PUSH

30 Days to **Turbocharged Habits,** a **Bangin' Body,** and the **Life You Deserve**

CHALENE JOHNSON

RODALE.

© 2012 by Chalene Johnson

No part of this publication may be reproduced or transmitted in any form or by any means,
electronic or mechanical, including photocopying, recording, or any other information storage
and retrieval system, without the written permission of the publisher.

Rodale books may be purchased for business or promotional use or for special sales.
For information, please write to:
Special Markets Department, Rodale, Inc., 733 Third Avenue, New York, NY 10017

Printed in the United States of America

Rodale Inc. makes every effort to use acid-free ☉, recycled paper ♾.

Photographs by Dan Mitchell
Family photos by Bosh Images
The TurboFire photo on page 74 is © Beachbody.com

Book design by Christopher Rhoads

Library of Congress Cataloging-in-Publication Data is on file with the publisher.

ISBN-10: 1–60961–333–3 hardcover
ISBN-13: 978–60961–333–4 hardcover

Distributed to the trade by Macmillan

2   4   6   8   10   9   7   5   3   1   hardcover

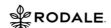

We inspire and enable people to improve their lives and the world around them.
www.rodalebooks.com

To Marge and Bill.

Dad, I know that you're reading
this to Mom from the throne where you read all your books.
Please tell Mom that I am forever grateful
that the two of you taught me how to be a devoted parent,
caring friend, loving spouse, and the best version of me.
I love you so much!

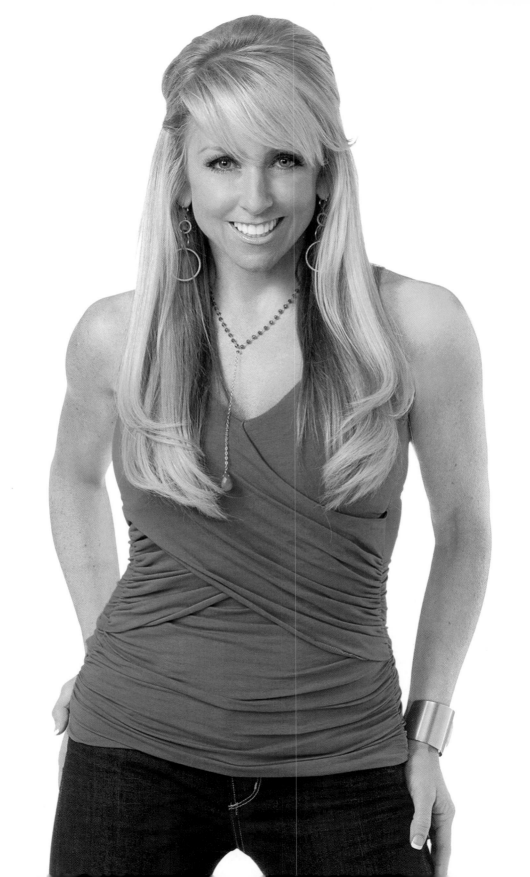

CONTENTS

PART 1: **THE 30-DAY PUSH**

PART 2: **3 CIRCUITS, ONE BANGIN' BODY!**

PART 3: **THROW-AND-GO RECIPES**

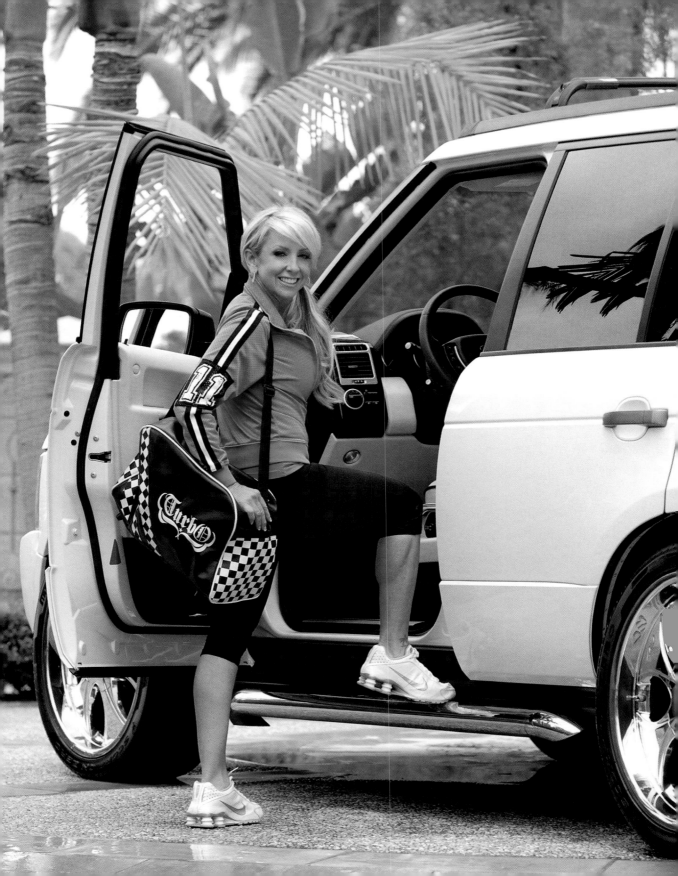

INTRODUCTION

As my husband and I walked to our car one day after my Turbo Kick class, he asked, "Why do you think that some of the people taking your class still have the same 20 pounds to lose that they had when they started 5 years ago, and others have completely transformed themselves and kept the weight off?"

Annoyed and feeling a bit responsible, I made it my mission to figure out what separated these two types of students.

After a few months of talking with people and observing them, I realized that the traits of the successful fitness enthusiasts had everything in common with those of the high achievers I had spent years studying in business. Accomplished, goal-mastering individuals live by the laws of success. It wasn't that their mind-set was so different or that they were of a particular genetic composition, displayed a specific intensity, or worked out more often.

What separated those who looked the same after 5 years from those who were able to transform their bodies and maintain their physique were merely their *habits*.

Health and Success Is a Matter of Habit

The solution has been in front of us all along. *Habits* are the key to success—routine behaviors so natural you don't need to give them much thought.

Successful people adopt the laws of success by creating lifelong habits that become ingrained and as much a part of who they are as the color of their eyes. They don't have to think about it. It's not torturous. It doesn't control their every conscious thought. It becomes second nature.

This book is about habits: how to break the bad ones and create the successful ones.

Plenty of diet books do an exceptional job of

teaching the principles of changing your mind-set, shifting your thinking, and altering the way you process information to help you change your body. Awesome books built on sound research. I love the idea of changing the way you think. But where most of these books fall short is that they miss what I have discovered to be the secret to long-term happiness and sustained weight management: the application of the laws of success.

The ingredients to lasting success in any area are universal, and one of the key ingredients is our consistent action. Those actions become our habits. Those habits change our thinking. Those habits change our body. Those habits define our destiny.

Habits have nothing to do with skill, financial position, education, appearance, or gifts from God. Anyone can learn to create a new habit. The right habits are the only things that separate you from the life you want to live.

It's very likely, however, that the life you currently *have* is making you fat. Oh sure, I can give you a great diet that, strictly followed, will allow you to drop megapounds, fast. If you want, feel free to skip the important stuff and jump into another diet. If you just love the roller-coaster diet and you think the stress lines across your forehead are quite attractive, well then, be my guest and skip the first 30-Day Push program in this book and go right to Part 2, the bangin' body workout. But if you do that, just know it'll be like sticking a Band-Aid on a bullet wound; another diet or a 30-day exercise program provides a temporary fix. But I think we've established that you're looking for a solution. Look no further.

Weight Isn't the Problem, Weight Loss Isn't the Solution

There are plenty of health experts out there prescribing lifestyles that *might* work if we lived in a utopian society where everyone gets 9 hours of sleep, receives massages once a week, and has a chef on staff, no kids, and 2 hours a day to spend in the gym.

Uh, hello! Reality check! I'm a crazy-busy devoted mom of two, I run several non-fitness-related businesses, and I enjoy date nights with my husband. I don't have a chef. We do have homework. There's always some kind of emergency, or dog poop to be picked up, and I have exactly 1 hour a day to exercise.

I live on this planet. I'm not going to freak out if on occasion you have a diet soda. Trust me, there are plenty of people who know more about exercise and nutrition than I do. The way that I have been of service to millions of people is by solving their health and fitness problems.

Your diet is a symptom. Your fitness or lack thereof is a symptom. They are not the problem, which is why addressing those areas as the solution provides only temporary relief.

I must admit that for the first 10 years of my career as a fitness professional, I too approached weight loss and fitness for my clients from this same dated perspective. I was stoked that my programs and diets worked for my clients but mystified when 6 months or a year later these folks ended up gaining the weight back or falling off the fitness wagon entirely.

Then it dawned on me. I was teaching them to drive a car without ever checking to see if they knew the rules of the road. Most would reach their destination, but eventually, when I handed over the wheel, they would crash.

That's why this book isn't a "It worked for me, it should work for you, too" approach. That's why I'm sharing the culmination of 2 decades' worth of interviews, studies, correspondences, follow-ups, medically supervised weight-loss and test groups, observations, and an exhaustive commitment to give you the best of what really works. A solution.

I've spent the past 20 years studying thousands of people. Listening, interviewing, tracking lasting success, understanding human nature, and unraveling the mystery of why some people diet all their lives and some make a permanent change. What I've learned is that you don't need another diet. You need a simplified way to organize your life. As a matter of fact, I am going to put your *life* on a diet so you can *stop* dieting once and for all.

How do you put your life on a diet? Well, I'm going to show you—day by day, one pain-free baby step at a time. I'm going to teach you how to quickly rebuild your foundation for success and identify where you want to go before we start your journey. I will share with you a "formula" to quickly discover which goals are right for you. This formula will allow you to set and master health and fitness goals that align perfectly with who you are and the life you want. I will teach you a few basic habits to restore balance, peace, happiness, and manageability to your supersize, chaotic life. Instead of dictating the perfect exercise pro-gram (which is kinda like an arranged marriage), I'll help you find your soul-mate workout, reach your fitness goals, blossom into a time management expert, become organized, and develop the tools to simplify difficult decisions.

PUSH will show you how to recognize toxic friends and separate from them without a big fat hairy confrontation. You'll learn how to deal with meddling family members, establish structure in your weekly routine, and find motivation in almost every area of your life.

I'll share with you the time-tested system I've used to help thousands of people not only reach their health and fitness goals but also learn how to live a more organized, purpose-driven, balanced life.

The Law of GYBIG (Get Your Butt in Gear!)

Oh, and . . . did I mention I like to start fires? Well, I do! So I plan to light a fire under your butt and then step back and fan the flames!

You're about to learn a focus and confidence you never knew you had, and through this process things are going to get better. Your thinking will begin to shift, your stress level will drop, your brain will change, your body will transform, and your life will gently sway into balance.

This book will do more than chisel your waistline; it will change the landscape of your life. Just a few days from now, people will smile, raise an eyebrow, and ask, "What has gotten into you? You're like a different person."

We'll start with a few choice habits. It's much easier to change your behavior than it is to change your genetics. It's also much easier to change behavior than it is to change thought patterns. In fact, it's much easier to change a few habits and create new behavior patterns than it is to change your brain. As they say, behave your way to success, and eventually your brain will follow. Experts suggest that married partners who have fallen out of love but who commit to behave as though they are deeply in love with their spouse will eventually experience a shift in their beliefs about their marriage.

I want you to know what works and what to do when it doesn't. You're a pretty smart cookie. You've figured out that a one-size approach to this problem doesn't solve much. We're individuals.

You want success, and you want it to last. Success is a matter of changing your routine and disciplining yourself to maintain a few well-proven habits. Period. Regardless of whether it's diet, business, relationships, fitness, parenting, or all of the above that have brought you to this book, if you adopt a few new habits, success is achievable. Best of all, once you rebuild your foundation with me in the first few chapters, the success you'll experience will trickle down into nearly every area of your life.

Your journey begins by learning the laws of success. The laws of success triumphantly apply to diet and exercise as they do to any other area of our lives. So before I give you the "perfect diet" or the "ultimate routine" (which we will get to, I promise), we need to start with a foundation.

Let's get started!

So while this is a "diet book," I want you to think of it as a lifestyle diet. I'd rather you adopt "a diet"—a way of living and eating that gives you joy. Really. Together, we will customize the way you'll nourish and strengthen your body for the rest of your life.

You're just about to learn the secret of how to do that. The truth is, it isn't a secret at all.

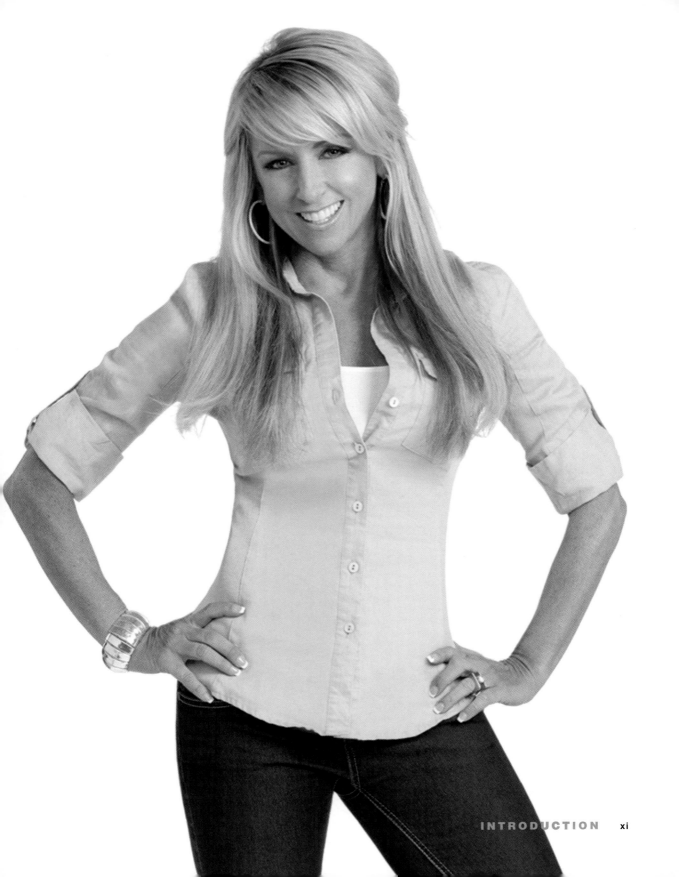

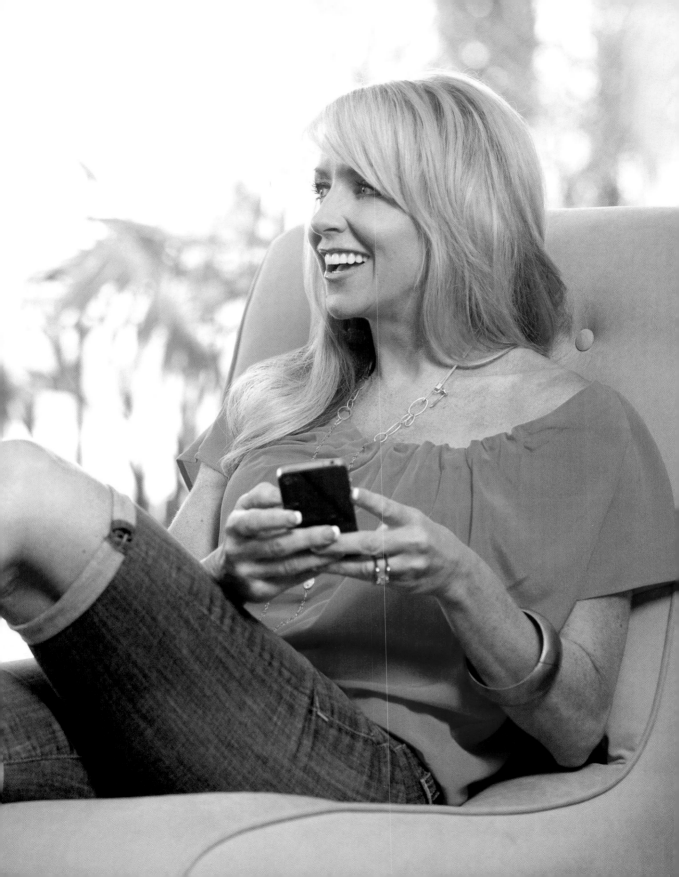

How to Make the Most of This Book

The cornerstone of all success begins with your foundation. By foundation, I mean the process of figuring out who you are, what's important to you, what gives you joy, what you want, and why you want it. When you build your life on bedrock, you stand tall, shoulders back, head up, smiling in the face of what might otherwise be a difficult decision, and just *know* what's right for you. You never wonder if you're doing the proper thing or if you're headed in the right direction.

Once you recognize your strengths and desires, you'll identify goals—both personal and physical—and analyze each for alignment with your priorities before you launch into action. As you learn basic time management and goal mastery, you'll be able to execute any plan with precision and live the life you deserve.

Heavy stuff—and stuff most people will never do. Successful people do what others know they should but will not. To become a success, or just to be *more* successful, you will do what average, less motivated people will not. Fewer than 30 days from now, you will have established the habits and foundation that the most suc-

cessful people on the planet share with you.

You're willing to spend 30 days with me as your "pusher" because you're supermotivated! *And* you're supersmart—smart enough to know that creating the life you deserve, and a bangin' body, to boot—is worth giving me the reins for the next 30 days.

Sure, you can skip ahead to the exercise and nutrition stuff and avoid the work of building your foundation. But if you give me just a few minutes a day, 30 days from now you can share the deeply ingrained habits of the most successful people on the planet.

It's your life. It's your health. It's your future.

You have dreams. You know you deserve more and that what you've done to this point has been average at best. You're no longer interested in average.

Once this foundation has been poured . . . oh, man . . . look out!

Your Foundation Determines Your Success

Whether you want a lasting marriage, a successful business, or a butt you can bounce a quarter off of, success requires a clear, well-engineered plan (along with discipline, action, and a clear idea of what we want, why, and what it'll take to get it). But while necessary, that plan is secondary; building a rock-solid foundation comes first. That plan needs to rest on *bedrock!*

I mean, we're all capable of creating and carrying out a plan. That's not too tough. In fact, that's how most small business and most diets begin, with a plan. Yet the plan provides no assurance of success. If it did, then 80 percent of all new businesses wouldn't fail within the first 5 years, and 85 to 90 percent of all dieters wouldn't gain their weight back in less than a year.

My point: Anything built to last—a house; a marriage; a successful, balanced, productive life—requires a strong foundation. So you need to get some things straight before you move to step two, the place where most diets and even most life plans begin.

You *reeeally* don't want to skip this crucial first step. Because just as homes crumble with-

out a strong foundation, people do, too. Those who lack strong foundations—a clear sense of who they are, what they value, their goals, knowledge of their strengths and weaknesses—struggle to find success in more areas than just their physical appearance or health. They wonder why, when they worked so hard to get things in place, once again life has tossed them upside down. Why don't things seem to work out for them the way they do for others?

The sad truth is, most people want a quick fix, and they're willing to try and try and try and just wing it. They're not willing to slow down and build a solid foundation once and for all. So even when the waters are calm, inside they're waiting for the storm to hit.

But that's not you. You get it. So you'll take the time to lay that foundation. Then not even the strongest gust can splinter your success. Lay that groundwork, and you'll no longer struggle with your weight and nutrition—or your relationships, finances, parenting, and work, for that matter. You'll experience lower levels of stress, less weight gain, fewer unexplained aches and pains or sleepless nights. You won't worry. You won't feel anxious.

Our foundations are often shaped as children and continue to form into adulthood. The good news is that you can fortify your foundation at any time. *Though it might be best just to knock the old one down and start from scratch.*

Most everything I'll teach you has been taught and practiced by the world's most successful personal productivity experts. I've simply adopted and simplified these techniques to work for your health, fitness, and diet—and I've had the pleasure of using the techniques to help others reach their goals, whether they have 10 or 100 pounds to lose.

Building a rock-solid foundation will give you the piece that has been missing in every diet book you've ever read. Am I right or am I right? No wonder even with a plan, most diets, businesses, and dreams never work out. They fail because they've left out a critical step!

Let Me Be Your Tech Support

Building a fit foundation is way easier than you think. It's kinda like trying to figure out your new phone without help or without reading the

Act Now and Receive a New and Improved Life—Absolutely *Free!*
No, you won't be getting a free set of kitchen knives or a blanket with sleeves, but the extra bonuses that come with this offer are so plentiful you would think it was too good to be true if I listed them.

You've probably already flipped through this book's table of contents and a few chapters and wondered what the heck making to-do lists and setting priorities have to do with losing weight. What are these things doing in a diet book?

Well, this "diet book" is different. Sure, it'll help you improve your health and your body—that's why you bought it. But it also holds out a bonus: the possibility of improvements in *all* areas of your life.

I think we can agree that to be healthy, both inside and out, you need balance. The cool thing about balance is that it's uniquely individual. How we spend our time and energy to create balance must be very personal.

Balance is possible only when you know how the scales should be set for you. Knowing how to balance your personal equilibrium comes only with full understanding of who you are, what gives you joy, and how you then execute the design of your life.

We've been led to believe that if we look "hot" or drive a certain car or wear a size 2, our life will fall perfectly into place. The truth is, when you strip all of it away, the one trait we all share is that we seek happiness.

We are the happiest when we feel worthy, deserving, accepted, and appreciated. We are the happiest when we are organized, confident, and know that we have the power to build and live the life we deserve.

While a rapid-start diet plan is awfully exciting, reread that last paragraph. Do you really think dropping a couple of pounds by Friday will lead you to long-term happiness? Sorry.

So try something different. Stop slapping a fresh coat of paint on the outside of a broken-down barn and let's do this right! Let's rebuild the foundation before we start building your new successfully happy, healthy, balanced life.

manual, versus sitting down with someone who already owns the phone and can accelerate your learning curve. Think of me as tech support for your fit-life foundation.

Together, we are about to build a fit foundation to create a healthy balanced life, and the task will be as painless as establishing a few new habits and developing some effective new skills. You'll soon see how my system works—and that it can improve *more* than your weight and health.

In our desire to be our best, lose weight, save money, find love, or get promoted, the likelihood of our success is boosted by the strength of our foundation. A fit foundation will give you confidence, assurance, and the self-love you need to stop looking outside yourself for acceptance. And this is where balance is found. Happiness is knowing who you are, what you want, and how you want it. Happiness is knowing you are doing the right things for yourself and the right people.

To build a fit foundation, you must first know who you are, what you want and don't want, and what you're not willing to compromise on. I'm talking about more than just your guiding principles or values. I mean your *priorities*. The exact life you would design if you had a magic wand, money wasn't an issue, and you had all the knowledge, skills, associations, and tools necessary to do this on your terms . . . the right way, the way *you* define "right way."

When you finish this book, you'll feel unstoppable. As I'm typing this, my heart is racing with the same excitement I have when the kids are rushing down the stairs on Christmas morning. Call me a geek, but I just get so pumped up for people to experience the control they have over their destiny by learning these really basic habits. I promise that 30 days from now you'll wonder why we didn't learn this stuff in school!

You've never done this before, and you're about to blow your own mind. This is crazy cool!

Make the Decision!

Today you lay the first brick of your foundation. That first brick? A decision.

You must decide that from now on, things will be different. That you're ready to change—not just for a day or a week, but for good. You must make a decision to succeed.

I had to make this decision, too. With obesity on both sides of my family, junk food a well-loved tradition in my household, and a physique topping out at 5 foot 2 inches, let's just say I had no choice but to figure out how I was going to maintain a healthy weight and positive body image and avoid the pitfalls of dieting. Well, I figured it out. Now I'm sharing my "secret" with you. And it begins with that decision.

This book is about how you can create successful habits and approach weight loss from the mind of a winner, a new person, someone committed to getting there once and for all. The totally cool part about this journey we're about to take is that it will actually help you to be more successful in all areas of your life. (Mark my words!)

So: Are you doing this or not? Are you in or are you out? Will you push or do you expect to be pulled? You've got 10 seconds to decide.

If you're willing to push, read on. If you're not sure, by all means, read on, but know that regardless of what chapter you're on, your journey starts with that decision. I can help you lose weight, but if you want to stop dieting and love your fit, balanced, and happy life, you have to believe it's forever. There must come a moment where you get over yourself and make a decision to do things differently.

Decide to Challenge That Inner Voice

Lasting success is powerfully tied to your beliefs. Your beliefs are also shaped by the conversations you're having all day long with others and, most powerfully, by the conversation you're having in your head—by the familiar sound of your inner voice.

What does yours sound like? What does it say? Do you hear:

You are a loser.

You're fat and the only chance you have of people liking you is if you get skinny.

Or do you hear a more encouraging voice:

Don't worry. You can do this.

You're going to crush it! You can do anything.

People don't care what size you are. People adore you and see you as healthy and fit.

The good news is that if you hear the first voice—the cruel, punishing voice that crushes your spirit—it can be silenced. Once you *decide* to succeed, that voice will be silenced.

Whether you believe you'll reach your goal and maintain a happy weight the rest of your life . . . or that you've just wasted your hard-earned money on yet another diet book, either way, you're right! Your mentality going in dictates your outcome.

While I was writing this book, a woman who had lost 95 pounds posted her story and a few before-and-after photos to my wall on Facebook. Hundreds of friends posted replies congratulating her. They praised her discipline and honored her inspiration.

One Facebook friend posted, "I've been overweight most of my life. This story is amazing! I only have 20 pounds to lose, but I doubt it will happen . . . even *with* one of your workouts, Chalene."

I replied to her post.

 Chalene Johnson Whether you believe you can lose the weight and keep it off forever or that it probably won't happen for you, either way, you're right! ☺

Moments later she replied "Message received loud and clear. Thanks for the much-needed wake-up call." Hundreds of similar replies like this one flooded my page:

 Malia Byron Thanks Chalene! Needed a dose of reality.

Whatever you believe about dieting, you're probably right. Whatever you believe about your abilities, your good luck or misfortune, your opportunities, the condition of your relationships, you're probably right!

Those who believe they can learn to manage their relationship with food, find their "soul mate" workout, and enjoy a life of health and fitness are *also* correct, and they have done so. Those who believe they can lose 100 pounds but worry that they will probably regain it are astutely correct.

Your beliefs are also shaped by your habits. What you believe about yourself shapes the course of your life! So along with swapping that negative inner voice for a more positive, powerful one, you must forge new, positive habits. I've got your back! I'll teach you to develop some very simple daily habits that will lead you to lasting success.

Decide to Ditch the Dieter's Mentality

Once you decide to succeed, you must give up thinking like a lifelong dieter. You gotta lose the dieter's mentality!

When you've been conditioned to adopt the dieter's mentality—and most women have been—you view "dieting" as a temporary prison sentence. You "cheat" with a "bad food" and then you get judged and punished . . . by yourself. Dieting is sort of like prison, isn't it? The same condemnation and judgment for bad behavior, followed by a period of punishment and deprivation.

And you can handle it . . . for a while! Until one day, life deals you an insane amount of crap and you just can't take it anymore. You rationalize that you're entitled to a cookie and you scarf it down. But you've just had the worst day ever. Screw it! You deserve another cookie! But *just one more.*

A sleeve of cookies later, you concede. You've blown it, just like you knew you would. You might as well enjoy that bag of chips and a few spoonfuls of ice cream at this point. Disgusted with yourself, you decide you'll start over, but you'll wait until after the upcoming vacation. You spend the next month gaining back the 8 pounds you lost plus 6 more from vacation gluttony. You're disappointed in yourself, unmotivated, and certain you'll never get off this roller coaster. (There's that negative inner voice again!)

Or maybe you've succeeded in losing those extra pounds. But if you have the dieter's mentality, you feel like your success is temporary. One day the jig will be up and everyone will know you're an imposter . . . a fat person masquerading as a thin one. So you keep your fat clothes, just in case.

Just in case? Just in case *what?* In case you fail?

"What if," "just in case," and "I'll try" are what you say when you believe failure is an option.

Bust out of that prison of shame and guilt—the one *you* built! You're a winner. From this day forward, success is your only option. It's the only choice you have. If I told you your family's life depended on your going the next 5 days with no food, no water, and no sleep, could you do it? Hell *yes,* you'd do it. Sit up straight, smile, and have the confidence of knowing you've already mastered the first step. You've just realized this whole thing hinges on your decision to *do* . . . not to try.

Decide to Succeed!

We all know the guy who's scheduled for this second bypass yet continues to smoke, drink, and eat crap, or the aunt diagnosed with type 2 diabetes who manages it with meds and lies to herself and everyone around her that she's changed her lifestyle. They both have beautiful kids or grandkids, great jobs, or whatever. Even with all of that at stake, it's not enough to motivate them to make a steadfast commitment to succeed.

If a life-threatening illness doesn't get your attention, what does? And that's the interesting part about my experiences with long-term successfully healthy folks.

All formerly unfit, unsuccessful people start their new life with a decision, a mental commitment, a day, a moment when they commit to live life differently—forever. I expected to find that for each of these people it was after a life-changing health scare, or hitting a certain number on the scale, but the catalysts of their decision were as varied as the individuals themselves.

For some it was a health scare, a photo, an all-time high on the scale, but for most it was a culmination of relatively tolerable events and their love for someone else that finally led to a moment of mental clarity in which they just decided *this must end!*

So while the decision must be yours, you may have heaped so much hate on yourself that right now you don't feel deserving of the transformation. It might be the love you have for someone else that brings you to this point.

But there's one thing I know: There's no transformation, no life changing, no bangin' body or better time management until you decide you are worth the effort.

So. No more excuses. No more hiding out. This is your moment. Make the decision to succeed. Once you do that—and believe me, that's the hardest part—success itself is just a few habits away. You'll never be the same person again.

Decided yet?

Come on. Do it now.

Did you make that decision? You *have?*

POOF!!! Failure has just been removed from your vocabulary. *Finito.* Gone. Success is yours to be had. You will soon have the tools and the habits to realize that with a solid plan, anything and everything is possible. By the time you finish this book, you will have put your life on a diet, put more food on your plate, have a bangin' body under cosnstruction, and developed a personalized plan for success that will trickle down into every nook and cranny of your life.

And it all began for you with that one decision: to succeed. From this moment on, nothing else that I ask you to do will be as difficult—or as exhilarating.

PART 1

The
30-DAY
PUSH

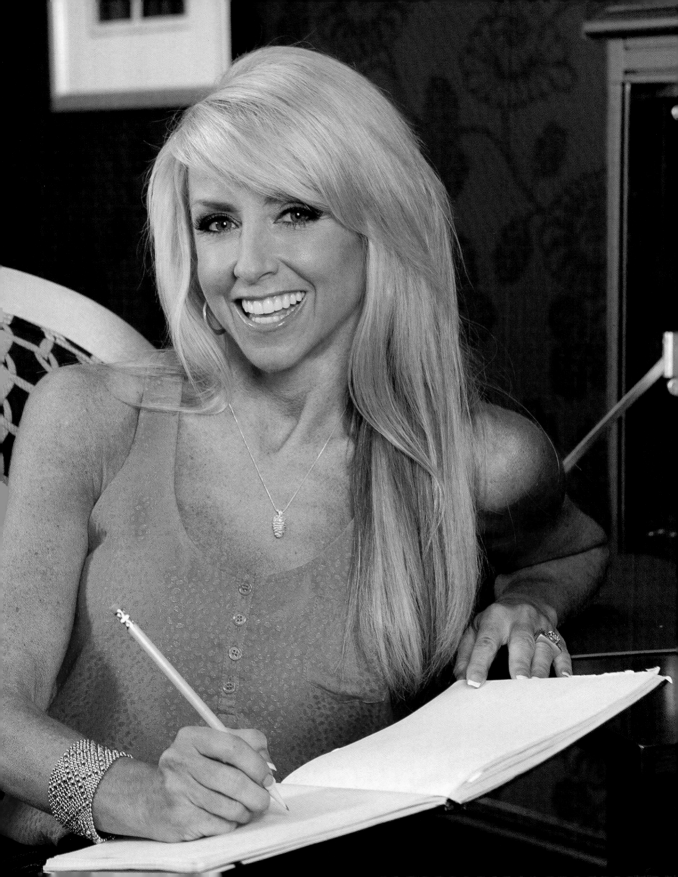

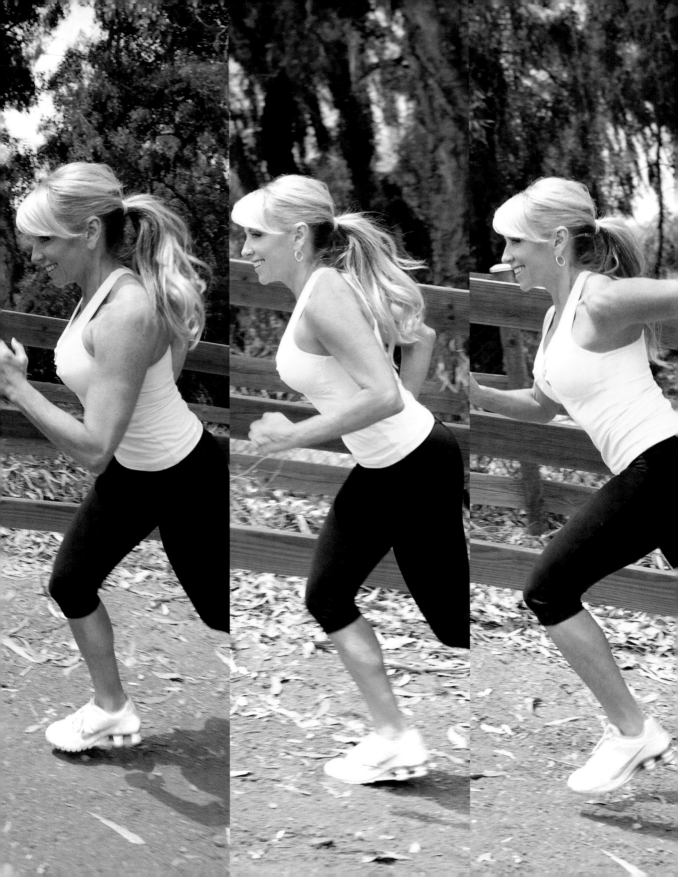

DAY 1
PRIORITIES
Defining What Matters Most

Tough stuff first. I'm not going to lie: The first day's assignment is the toughest and the most important. The good news is this is also the most important day of this challenge. The work you'll do today will influence every area of your life for the rest of your life.

Mastering goals is simple. Anyone can do that. And plenty of people do, only to find they've arrived but feel lost, lonely, deeply dissatisfied, and living a life devoid of balance.

What Day 1 of the Push Plan teaches you to do is *identify* your goals. That takes more thought, more reflection, more work. But don't stress. I'm here to lead you through the process, and you won't believe how much more focused and energized you'll feel once it's done!

Lessons from a Toddler's Toy

We all know the Shape-O Toy—that bright red, blue, and yellow plastic ball that teaches little kids their shapes. Either we had one or we got one for our kids. The Shape-O ball comes with 10 plastic shape pieces—a star, a circle, a triangle, and so on—that the child pushes through openings in the ball that are the same shape as the pieces.

The toddlers select a piece and then press it against the opening they believe the piece will fit through. No matter how much they push and turn the shape, the star piece won't fit through the circle hole, right? The square piece won't fit into the opening made for a triangle. And so on—the pieces simply won't "fit" until they're pressed against the right opening in the ball.

But by the time you're 3, you've figured out you can cheat! Pull on the ball's yellow handles, and the ball splits in half, allowing you to shove anything you want into the center.

Unfortunately, that's how most people decide if a goal or an opportunity, or even a mate, is a good fit. They *make* it fit. But alas, sometimes they "cheat"—and who they're cheating is themselves!

Wouldn't it be great if you had a simple tool, like a Shape-O ball, to know if something was going to be the right fit (she asked excitedly, knowing there *is* such a tool!).

The first step in reaching your goals is setting ones that are a good fit. Whether you focus on health and fitness, business, marriage, faith, or parenting, before you set goals, you need to have a better system of identifying which ones will fit.

Call them your defining values, your principles, call 'em what you want, but for our purposes we're going to call them your "life priorities."

So many people set and achieve goals only to find they're no happier than when they started. That's because most people never take the time to sit down and figure out who they are and what's really important. In other words, they never create those shapes on the outside of a Shape-O ball, so they have nothing to press against.

Intrinsic Priorities

I define intrinsic priorities as areas of critical importance so ingrained into who you are that you really need no accountability to honor their place. In other words, these intrinsic priorities don't even need to go on your life priorities list. You honor them naturally.

For example, you might be surprised to know that health and fitness don't go on my formal life priorities list. My hope is that health and fitness at some point in your near future become intrinsic priorities.

I did this priorities exercise with a small group of business professionals, many of whom also happen to be devout Christians. Only one listed "faith" in the top three priorities. When I questioned the others about their decision to leave their faith off the list, one member rather confidently replied, "You know, it's such a part of who I am, I didn't even think to put it in the list."

Perfect! Certain intrinsic priorities have become a part of your fabric. Being a kind person, working to treat people with fairness, those things are intrinsic priorities. I feel as though I need no accountability. I'm perfectly happy with the amount of attention I give this area. No more. No less. So if your intrinsic priorities are who you are, the balance is just right and you already live according to that priority. It doesn't need to go on your list.

But say, for example, building your business is something that is important to you but you need to give it more energy and time, then you are not living according to your top priority, and building your business needs to go on your list. Intrinsic priorities are part of your fiber, a part of who you are.

In the worksheet below, you will write out your priorities, what's important to you, the compass by which you direct your life, your values, what gives you joy, what gives you purpose, what gives you pride. Understanding your priorities is the first step in restoring life balance.

PRIORITIES: THE SHAPE-O BALL EXERCISE

Only when you know what (and who) is most important, with clarity, should you set goals and take action. To truly be successful, you need to match your goals with your personal priorities.

Clearly defined priorities allow you to easily identify your most effective use of time and your most valiant pursuits, thus simplifying life's toughest decisions. Once you've identified your priorities, you've, in essence, created a Shape-O ball for your life.

Say your number-one priority is to be actively engaged and to spend more time with your family, or maybe you want to devote additional hours at work to get that promotion. In that case, setting a goal to win a fitness competition is a poor choice. No matter how hard you push the goal of "9 percent body fat" against your Shape-O ball, it will never converge with your most important current life priorities.

You're seconds from starting an exercise that will allow you to quickly match up your goals and immediately know if they fit. To get the most from it, you need to write it on paper and not just in your head. Know how your goal is going to fit before you pursue it.

Believe me, this exercise works. I recently spoke to a group of insurance executives and took them through the process—actually made them write it out, as you will. After my speech, one of their top-level professionals approached me, a big smile on his face.

"I just have to tell you," he said, stunned but excited. "That exercise helped me make a decision I've been struggling with for more than 10 years. I've been chasing the wrong dream, and I never really understood that until today, when you had us write out this exercise."

He went on to explain that he was being held prisoner by a high-paying career that gave him no joy and kept him from his family. He worked long hours, sometimes 7 days a week, and the trappings of money combined with the distance between him and his family had created a lot of unhappiness.

Later, I found out he had quit his high-paying career to become a professor of music. I don't know him personally, but I'd bet my life savings he's living a more balanced life!

How My Homework Helped Me

Every person who has completed the priorities homework and created a top priority clarity statement has told me the process has given them the tools to revisit long-standing tough decisions, reevaluate their path, and gain the confidence they needed to know they were making the right decision.

It's sure worked for me. Let me give you an example from my own life. My mission has always been to solve problems for people: to help people find a way to live balanced, fit, successful lives and to place the greatest amount of energy on our relationships.

To share this message on a national level without impacting my number-one priority meant I had to be creative. Infomercials were the perfect fit. Not easy to get into the business, true; but nothing worth having ever is easy. I knew success in the infomercial arena would

(continued on page 10)

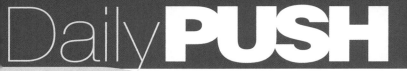

Today's Homework

PRIORITIES

This little exercise has changed the lives, career paths, and fitness journeys of thousands. Read today's assignment undistracted. Grab a pencil and paper. We'll transfer this information to your smartphone, but your best thinking is done old-school style—with a sharpened No. 2 pencil and a crisp piece of paper.

Start by brainstorming your priorities. Use the space below (or better yet, create a dedicated PUSH journal so you have even more space if you need it) to list any and all areas of importance in your life today. Priorities are those things that are so important that if they were stripped from your life, you would be devastated, unfulfilled, and living without purpose. Who do you want to be? What do *you* want to accomplish? What makes *you* happy? What do you think is your purpose in this life? What gives *you* pride? What do you wish to be remembered for at the end of your life? What do you want people to know was most important to you? What makes you feel good about yourself? What areas of your life are of great importance *yet* you believe you must keep yourself accountable to honor them?

_____

_____

_____

_____

Place a star next to the five areas that are most important to you.

Now list the three priorities (in no particular order) that you have identified as most important to you. Use just a few words to identify each category, such as "faith," "family," "career," "my charity," "my health," and so on.

_____

_____

_____

_____

▶ Rewrite the list in order of importance to you:

My number-one priority: _____

My second priority: _____

My third priority: _____

▶ Take the priority you've listed as number one and complete the following statements:

▶ The reason(s) I have placed the greatest importance on this area of my life is because:

_____

_____

▶ I will honor my number-one priority by doing my best to:

_____

_____

▶ The following action(s) would be inconsistent with my commitment to my top priority:

_____

_____

▶ To honor my number-one priority, I will limit the following:

_____

_____

▶ To honor my number-one priority, I need to make the following changes:

_____

_____

▶ Now you're ready for the last question on the worksheet—and it's so important it gets its own section.

Creating Your Top Priority Statement

With as much detail as possible, create a "top priority clarity statement" in the space below. Here are some examples.

My number-one priority is to fortify and honor my relationship with my family by spending more time together, listening, engaging, and sacrificing to help each member feel important, admired, trusted, respected, and supported in our everyday lives and to limit activities and pursuits that might be harmful to these relationships.

My number-one priority is to build my business by being present, disciplined, and focused on serving my customers and committing to learning everything I can about leadership, management, and business success and eliminating excuses, distractions, and unproductive pursuits.

▶ Here's my own top priority clarity statement:

My number-one priority is to be present and actively involved in the lives of my husband and children; to demonstrate through my actions that my children are more important than any personal pursuit; to work to strengthen my loving, respectful, and supportive relationship with my husband as a means to provide the best possible environment for my family; to raise self-sufficient, confident children who believe they can do anything; to limit any activities, pursuits, or relationships that might take me away from my family; and to weigh all decisions against what would be helpful, harmful, or indifferent to my family's emotional well-being.

▶ Now write yours. Take all the time you need.

_____

_____

_____

_____

_____

_____

▶ Write or print out your top priority clarity statement and post it on your computer, near your desk, in your kitchen, on the inside of your medicine cabinet, and, hey, why not make it the lock screen on your smartphone? Memorize it. With this statement front and center, it's miraculous how clear even the toughest decisions become.

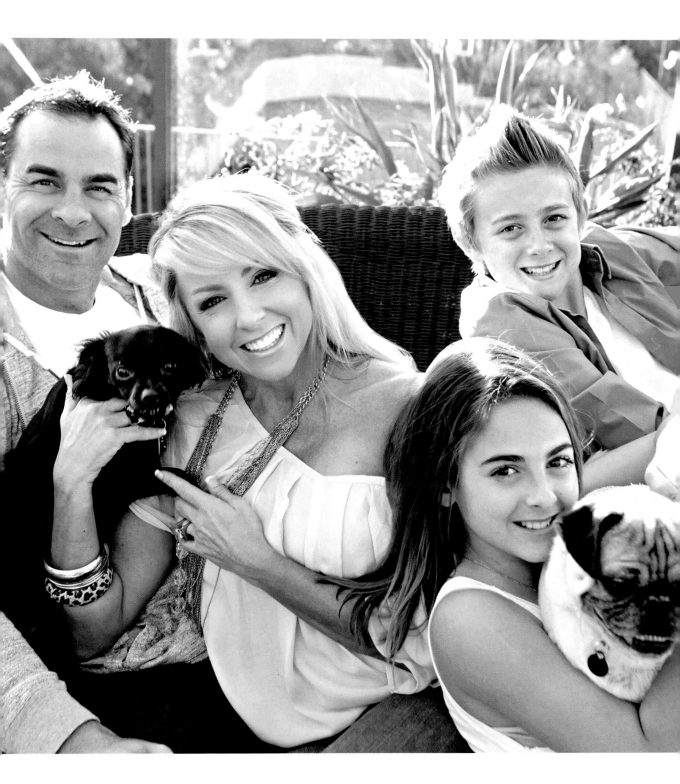

allow me a degree of anonymity (even though I've sold millions and millions of exercise DVDs, no one really recognizes me), so this means the kids can lead a normal life. I can go to the mall or the grocery store. It's cool. The high volume of sales allows me to provide for my family in a way that enables me to be home most of the time, work from my home office, control my own schedule, and take a ton of vacations.

But when a great opportunity presented itself at a time when I was less financially secure, I had to weigh the decision against my top priority clarity statement.

In one of those periods of financial weakness, I got a call from a producer of a prime-time weight-loss competition show. The producer had seen my work and was interested in speaking to me about the possibility of filling one of the trainer spots for the upcoming season. Even though the opportunity would have helped my brand and probably in the long run made me millions more in endorsements and notoriety, in my evaluation it didn't fit with any part of my top priority clarity statement.

I politely declined and thanked him for thinking of me.

Silence. Then he said, "I'm not sure if you heard me correctly, this is for [insert name of Very Big Show About Losing Weight here]."

Now, had I not clearly defined my priorities years prior, I would have second-guessed my decision. I would have wondered if I had made the biggest mistake of my career. Instead, because I knew my priorities, it was an easy decision.

Without a clear top priority statement, I would have just thought in my head, *Well, my family is my first priority, and this opportunity will allow me to better provide for them, and it's a once-in-a-lifetime op, so take it.* But because I had created a clearly defined statement, I was able to quickly make what for other people would have been a very difficult decision.

I understood what he was saying. I didn't feel a moment of indecision. There was no "what if" or even a phone call to run the scenario by my husband, Bret. We are very clear about what is most important and how we have defined that. Being a present force in my children's day-to-day life would not have been an option if I had taken the offer.

When people say to you, "I don't know if another opportunity like this is going to come your way!" you tell them, "I don't need one to come my way. I am smart enough and motivated by my priorities. I won't wait for opportunities; I will create those that fit me."

You are resourceful. You're smart. You deserve the life you want, but it doesn't just "come around." You have to plan for it. Take action and keep at it. Sure, it might take longer to do it "right," but nothing beats the pride you'll have by doing it properly.

Something better, something that fits perfectly into your Shape-O ball, will come your way—and if it doesn't, you'll create it! Let's start creating right now.

Think about these questions as we move along to the next chapter. What do you want to feel like 12 months from now? How much would you like to weigh? How fit will you be? How many days per week will you be exercising? How much time will you be vacationing? How much money would you like to earn? Twelve months from now, if the stars were perfectly aligned, what crazy, outlandishly cool things would you like to see happen?

It's a lot to think about. Just going through the questions in this chapter are all the work you need to do today. I suspect your brain is on overload—in a good way! It's kinda like the first day back to school when the teacher hands you the course syllabus but gleefully announces there will be no homework that night.

From tomorrow forward, consider yourself an honor student, and prepare yourself mentally to take on just a few quick assignments each day. I call these tasks your Daily Push. Remember, I would never dream of pushing you unless I thought you were up for the challenge and deserved the rewards.

DAY 2
GOAL SETTING

"Wouldn't It Be Crazy Cool If . . . "

Now that you've completed your first assignment, we get to do the fun stuff. You've got your three life priorities. You know how you're going to honor them. You're now going to learn how to quickly set and accomplish goals that are aligned with your priorities and consistent with the things that are most important to you.

The vital difference between dreamers and achievers boils down to some very basic, simple habits. People with clear, *written-out* goals who consistently honor their defined priorities tend to get results faster than others and enjoy a greater level of happiness and long-term success in all areas of life. Yet most of us have never been formally taught a system of goal setting and mastery that can be applied to health and fitness.

By learning the most effective ways to set and attain your goals, you will be able to achieve your health and fitness goals faster than you ever dreamed possible and reduce a major amount of stress. More important, your results will last a lifetime.

In my own experience, learning to set goals and stay on task by using a daily to-do list (sneak preview of what's coming to a chapter near you) changed my life. When you learn how to set goals aligned with your priorities and execute them with the convenience of a text message, you soon recognize that absolutely anything you envision for yourself is possible. In this chapter, I will teach you the skill of setting and attaining your goals with basic simplicity rather than just letting all of these ideas bounce around in your head.

Goals must move from your brain to a page. So consider this moving day! Written goals give us clarity and direction. Desires or thoughts such as "I wish I could fit into those jeans again!"

or "I'm going to get my butt in shape for summer!" are often mistaken for goals. Goals give us a specific destination to focus our actions and energies. Written goals help you to better communicate to others, as well as to yourself, your plans for the future. Goals relieve stress and bring clarity to your starting point. Written goals provide motivation and accountability that far surpass "thought bubble" goals or even spoken goals without measurements or deadlines.

Mission Possible: 10 Goals a Week

For the next 28 days, your assignment is to create a list of 10 goals once a week. At least one of them should relate to your health. You'll write your first 10 goals today. So whatever day you're reading this, mark your calendar—7 days from right now, you're going to create another list of 10 goals.

Today your mission is to come up with a list of 10 things that will be so flipping cool when they happen in the next year. That's how I want you to think about it. Don't think that any event or achievement is impossible, crazy, or out of the realm of possibility. I just want you to think, "Wow, wouldn't it be crazy cool if this happened?" And write it down. Things you want to have happen. Things you're dreaming of happening. Things you will *make sure* happen.

Don't set goals you know you're going to accomplish—for example, "Twelve months from now, I hope to be a little bit more successful." *Helllllooo*—that goal is a done deal! Nope, I want you to set goals for yourself that are *tough*. This is a challenge. You've already committed yourself to this, and your challenge is to come up with 10 wonderfully challenging goals. And here's how I want you to think of it:

Ten goals that if everything is perfectly aligned, if you have all the financing, all the schooling, all the education, all the right opportunities, if the stars were perfectly aligned, you will make possible in 12 months. Just brainstorm—take out a piece of paper and start writing. What's crazy about this is that many of you will probably get to number five or six and then you'll really have to think. It's like, "Wow, what else do I want?" So let me give you some ideas to get you through that writer's block.

When you think of your goals, think of financial goals, goals you have for your relationships, your happiness, how you want to spend your time, personal goals you have for yourself—do you want to become more organized, do you want to pay off a car loan, do you want to have your business reach a certain financial status? Just keep thinking about what else you can come up with.

Now, what should *not* go on your list is anything that relates to something you have no control over. So, for example, I can't say that I have a goal for my husband because he's the only person in charge of that. I can't say that my kids are going to get straight A's because really, that's up to them. So you want to set goals over which you have total control. And trust me, as we move through the next couple of days, you're going to realize how incredible this opportunity is because it's just about creating a habit. Once you've set your goals for yourself, then you're going to start to tackle them.

Now let's do it!

Guidelines for Goal Setting

You're just about ready to set your goals—get that pencil ready! But before you start, I want to give you some guidelines that will help you complete the homework below.

YOUR GOALS SHOULD MESH WITH YOUR PRIORITIES *All* of them. Ask yourself if the goal could compromise one or all of your priorities. If so, is there a way to accomplish nearly the same result in a creative way that doesn't compromise your priorities?

YOUR GOALS SHOULD BE PERSONAL AND PROFESSIONAL Consider relationships, finances, health, faith, hobbies, habits, leisure pursuits, anything that comes to mind. The sky's the limit.

YOUR GOALS SHOULD TAKE YOU OUT OF YOUR COMFORT ZONE Don't list goals you already know you've achieved or that you're well on your way to achieving. No easy stuff. I want 10 goals that are an uncomfortable stretch but in the realm of possibilities.

IF YOU GET STUCK, COMPLETE THIS SENTENCE When it seems you've run out of ideas and you need inspiration, use the following statement, "In the next 12 months, it would be so crazy cool if _____."

WRITE YOUR GOALS IN THE PRESENT TENSE Write your goals as if they have already been achieved, speaking in the first person and with as much detail as possible, such as "I am a *New York Times* best-selling author."

INCLUDE GOALS THAT PUSH YOU TO MAKE PERSONAL CHANGE Goals can address areas of personal improvement, such as: "I am seeking treatment for my eating disorder and will weigh myself only once a month."

INCLUDE AT LEAST ONE FINANCIAL GOAL Most everything you want in life, from having more time off, paying off your home, and helping others to having more time for exercise, is made easier with financial means. Money issues are one of the top causes of personal stress, which you already know may be the number-one thing standing between you and your new lean body. Therefore, at least one of your goals needs to relate to finances.

LIST ONE HEALTH GOAL WITH A VERY SPECIFIC MEASURE For example, "I have lost over 40 pounds and I have cut my body fat in half." A downloadable PDF version of this form is available free for you at www.chalenejohnson.com/goals-worksheet. Download this form and give it to the important people in your life to set some goals with you! You can also go directly to the digital version so that it can be done from your smartphone: www.chalenejohnson.com/digitalGoalworksheet.

Now it is time to go all out and do some goal setting!

Why Once a Week?

You may be wondering why I want you to create a new list of goals each week. Well, there's a very good reason: The exercise of rewriting them once a week acts as a filter that in the end reveals what truly is important to you: your real hopes and dreams, your authentic vision for your future.

Every time you set your goals and write them down on paper, it's like they solidify in your brain. Even setting goals once a year is pretty

(continued on page 18)

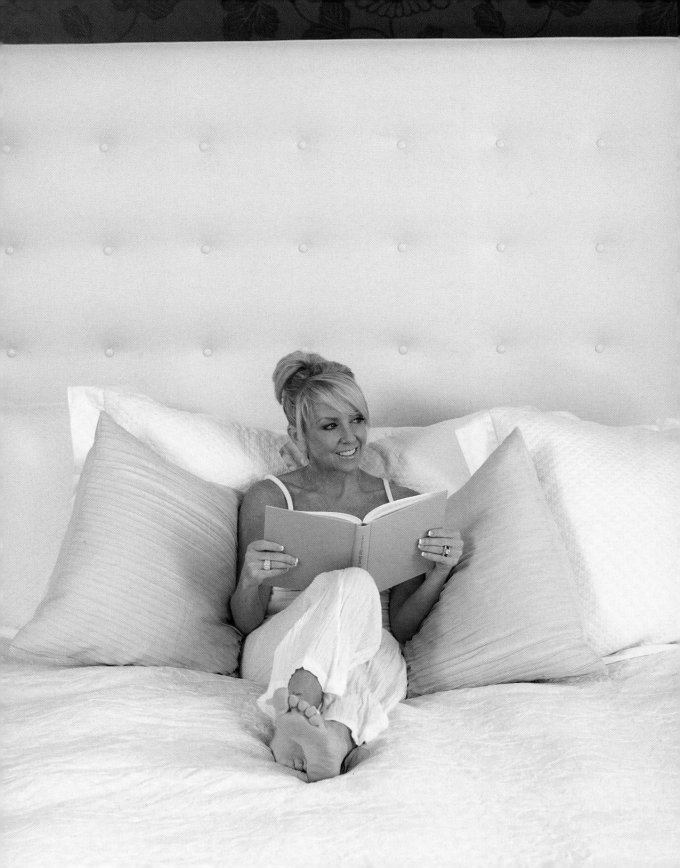

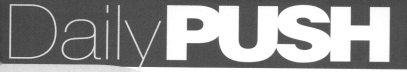

Homework

GOAL SETTING

The goals you set should be things that, when you achieve them, you're going to be over-the-moon proud! They take work, but they're exciting enough that you're motivated to put in the sweat equity.

Think about the 10 things that you would love to see happen—financial, physical, personal, from a business standpoint, from a spiritual standpoint, from a relationship standpoint, anything that you can think of—12 months from now. (I told you this would be fun!)

Just list your top 10 goals. Leave your Push goal and your health goal blank for now. We will identify them in Days 3 and 4.

GOALS!   Date_____

Push goal: _____

Health goal: _____

1. _____

2. _____

3. _____

4. _____

5. _____

6. _____

7. _____

8. _____

9. _____

10. _____

So let's take a look at your list of 10 goals. As you read over each one, ask yourself:

Is each goal specific? "I want to be thin" is too vague. Give it a measure: a size, a body-fat percentage, a specific range—something that can be quantified.

Specifics give you confidence, keep you accountable, and hold your feet to the fire. "I am making more money" and "I have paid off some of my debt" are way too easy and too vague for someone like you—someone who is going to kick ass in the next 12 months!

Do I believe I can accomplish this goal the next 12 months? When you set goals that are vague, such as "improve health," you never really experience the satisfaction that comes with checking something off your list. Pointing to one of the numbers on your goal list and saying proudly, "Wow! I did it!" feels pretty darned amazing. I want you to set goals so cool that you can't wait to tackle them.

Could I dream even bigger? Don't be afraid to hope. Go big! When I did this goal worksheet with my best friend in the spring of 2010, she listed that she wanted to earn $500,000 with her home business. I said, "What?! No way! I know you. I know your passion and how organized and committed you are to growing your business. I also know you're already on your way to hitting that financial goal. So what you're saying is you hope you can maintain that momentum? No way, Monica. What's a number that would be really exciting, but really tough? The kind of number that means getting focused?" She said, "Well, I guess to be earning $15,000 a week would be crazy cool."

A year later, guess what she was earning? Yup! And hitting that financial goal allowed her to fulfill most of the other numbers on her list. Her husband retired from his full-time career to work side by side with her helping other couples navigate the waters of running a business together. With www.partnerwithyourpartner.com, she learned to snowboard, took eight vacations, cut back on her personal training clients so she was home more often, hired a personal assistant, spent more time with her family, and, most important, she created a far less stressful and far more balanced life for her husband and their triplets. (Yes, you read that correctly. Parents with triplets are living a balanced, low-stress life? Yup, and you can, too!)

I tell you this story because it drives home an important point: Somewhere along the way, people lose belief in themselves. They forget that they too deserve the possibility of a perfectly designed life.

So let me push you. Pretend right now that you and I are looking at your goals together. Would you be able to say your goals are very challenging? Are you stretching yourself? Will your goals require you to do things differently? Do they push the status quo? If you don't aspire toward greatness, you cannot achieve greatness. It's really that simple. And if you aspire toward small things, you will achieve small things. Sure, you can set your goal to be "I want to organize my closet." And I bet you'll actually achieve it. But, we're talking about setting some jump-off-the-cliff, this-is-scary-but-I-can-do-it kind of goals!

Once you've listed your goals, asked yourself those three questions, and are satisfied that each and every one of the 10 goals you listed is both doable *and* crazy cool, go back and ink 'em. That's right. Write them in ink. There! You're committed now.

powerful, and I did that for many, many years.

But when I started doing it once a week—holy cow! Insanity! Each time you rewrite your goals, you intensify their power. At first I'd blow through the goals on my list in 12 months. Eventually, though, I started blowing through them in 4 or 5 months—6 months, at the most—and I'd have to create new goals.

So *that's* why I want you to set goals once a week.

Here's the caveat: I don't want you to look back at the goals you wrote the week (or weeks) before, because I want those goals, and the process, to be organic. What you'll find at the end of our challenge is that each week—especially if you don't cheat—probably five or six of those items will stay the same and four, maybe two or three, it just depends, will change. You'll begin to see a pattern, and from that pattern you'll be able to identify which goals are most important.

Daily PUSH

1. Complete your list of 10 goals as outlined in this chapter.

2. Transfer that list of goals to a place for safekeeping: a journal, your smartphone, or your desktop.

NOTES

_____

_____

_____

_____

_____

_____

_____

_____

The Smartphone Advantage

For hundreds of years, writing out goals has been taught as one of the pillars of success. And it always will be. But if you have a smartphone, you can turbocharge the speed at which you achieve your goals and give goal setting a 21st-century makeover.

Earl Nightingale, whom many considered to be the dean of personal development, once said that we become what we think about most. Now, because of technology, we have this incredible advantage. In the past, before the use of smartphones, if you wanted to think about something, if you needed to focus your thoughts around your goals, you had to rely on your memory. I don't know about you, but my memory is out of hard drive space. Not too reliable. Thank goodness for my phone!

When it comes to weight training, I'm fanatical about proper technique. My personal training clients used to call me a "freak for form." I'm equally passionate about smartphones. Call me a cell snob if you must, but my persistence stems from a sincere belief that if it makes life easier for people, I have a duty to push. Now listen, there are plenty of very smart people who do not have smartphones. You might be one of them. Most people who don't use a smartphone say, "I just don't know why I would need one." I get it. It's hard to imagine *needing* something you've gone this long in life without. I remember thinking the same thing about the Internet. Today, I can't imagine how we survived before Wi-Fi.

Of course you'll survive without a smartphone. Your success does not hinge on whether you have a digital device. BUT . . . it will give you an edge. It will make life easier. Your smartphone becomes your personal trainer, your accountability, and your personal assistant in your pocket.

Some technologies you can do without. I happen to believe the smartphone is one of the game-changing breakthroughs that can have a tangible impact on every corner of your life. You don't have to make a decision today. You can get where you're going without it. I just ask that you keep an open mind. It's an investment that I promise will pay you dividends.

Identifying Your
PUSH GOAL

What One *Goal Helps You Achieve All the Others?*

You have spent the past two days soul searching and making lists. Today, it's time to start making things happen. Now that you've completed your list of 10 crazy cool things you would love to see happen in the next 12 months, all of which are consistent with your top three priorities, you're going to identify your Push goal and your health goal. Today, we'll focus on your Push goal!

The Push Goal: The Domino Effect

You know how when you set up a stack of dominoes in a line, very close to one another, and then push the first one gently with your finger? What happens? The action of that first domino topples all the others. And that's the best way to think of your Push goal: It's that first domino!

I developed the concept of the Push goal after 15 years of working as a coach and business advisor. It was my response to a tendency I'd observed in even the most goal-oriented individuals: After they'd set their 10 personal goals for the year, they often didn't know which goal to tackle first. So generally, they'd start with the easiest to accomplish.

Just one problem: The easiest goal tended to result in the least rewarding outcome, which diminished their personal mojo. I saw people losing motivation and interest, even when their top 10 goals were in writing.

To identify the problem, I analyzed my clients' lists of goals—and noticed that there was always one goal which, once achieved, would make possible or "push through" the other goals. Voilà! The Push goal was born.

Let me give you an example, from my own life, of how to identify your Push goal. Here's my list of 10 goals from March 2010. (As I taught you in Day 2, I wrote my goals in the present tense, first person, as if I'd already achieved them.)

Daily PUSH

1. Refer to the goals worksheet from Day 2 and identify which of the 10 is your Push goal.

2. Write your Push goal across the top of your goals worksheet, print, and post!

3. Share your goals list with a wise friend or companion who can confirm that you've chosen the right Push goal or at least offer his or her valued feedback.

NOTES

_____

_____

_____

_____

_____

_____

_____

1. I am a *New York Times* best-selling author.

2. I am enjoying 8 weeks of vacation with my family.

3. I mentor a team of new entrepreneurs on a weekly basis.

4. I offer a free 30-day course that I created to teach productivity and goal mastery.

5. One hundred thousand people take advantage of my free 30-day course.

6. I conduct four life-changing seminars, two of which I share the stage with industry mentors like Brendon Burchard and Brian Tracy.

7. I devote a special day each week to each of my children, where we do one-on-one activities.

8. I plan surprise dates and mini-vacations for my husband.

9. I am sharing my message of life balance on things like time management, relationships, delegating, etc., through a series of monthly training programs on CD or audio download.

10. I am 12 months without an injury that limits my fitness regimen.

I identified my Push goal as number 5. Here's how I did it.

When I made this list, I knew that the most important goals for me were those related to Bret or the kids. Yet, I also knew that *some of my professional goals could make those personal goals easier to achieve.*

Let me explain my thinking. If I have more Internet notoriety, more people will buy my audio and video training programs. When I can help people and share my message without having to travel away from my family, I honor my number-one priority. The best way to achieve that notoriety without doing a prime-time TV show or another project that might take me away from the kids is to have a book reach number-one status on the *New York Times* best-seller list.

In researching what it takes to reach *NYT* bestseller status, I learned that it entails more than a great book or a big fan base. It requires a trusting and loyal base of customers who you have helped and who are eager for your book. It takes promotion and planning.

Therefore, the goal on my list that makes *NYT* bestseller status possible is number 5— having 100,000 people go through my 30-day productivity course. If I can help 100,000 people live more organized lives, they will have a track record with me. They will want to buy the book. I will have established a relationship with them outside of being their exercise guru. That relationship also makes my brand more attractive to personal development greats like Brendon Burchard and Brian Tracy. Therefore, the free 30-day course (which I *did* create in 2010 and set up at www.30daypush.com) helped me to achieve goals 1, 3, 4, 6, and 9. Achieving goals 1, 3, 4, 6, and 9 makes all the others on the list possible.

In other words, goal 5 became the catalyst for every other goal on my list.

That's the kind of reasoning I want you to use as you try to identify your personal Push goal. It's an exercise in reasoning.

Today's Homework

IDENTIFYING YOUR PUSH GOAL

Turn back to Day 2, analyze your list of 10 personal goals, and decide which is your Push goal. It's not necessarily the goal that's the most important to you but *the one that makes all the others possible*.

Are you undecided between two goals? Don't stress. That happens sometimes, that you have two goals that seem to have equal potential. Ask yourself which goal leads to the path of least resistance. That is your Push goal. If you still can't decide, just pick one for now. You can reevaluate as we go.

Fill in the Push goal line on your goals worksheet from Day 2.

Now evaluate your Push goal. Is it a skill or is it measurable? Does it challenge you enough? Let's revisit my 100,000-people Push. It's measurable— I've attached a number to it, I've attached a date. I can measure how well I'm doing based on how many people are taking this particular challenge. As for whether it is challenging enough, there are many skills I have to learn or master, which I figured out when I did my brainstorm. So ponder your list— you'll find the answers you're looking for.

We're all a work in progress. There is no failing in this process. You're learning, you're deciding, you're researching. And every day you do that, your brain just expands, and it's exciting because you realize what type of potential you have. But I want to make sure that you set a Push goal that will challenge you, that will make you feel like the queen of the world when you accomplish it.

Yes, there are skills you must master to reach that goal. Add those skills to a list of to-dos, things you must accomplish, but don't make those skills your Push goal.

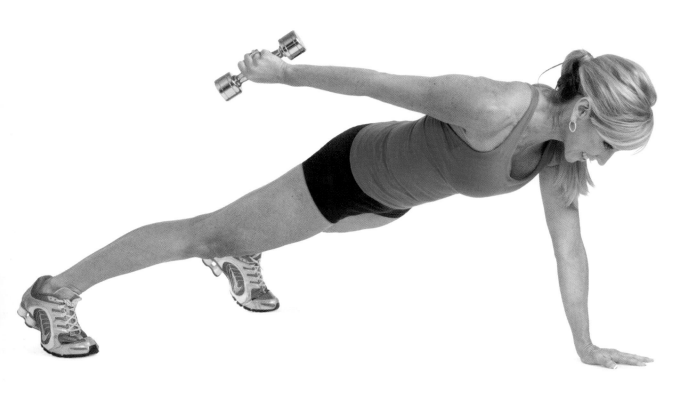

Selecting a SMART HEALTH and FITNESS GOAL

Getting Smart about Getting Lean

Not too many years ago, a middle-aged woman with a thick midsection and a friendly smile walked into one of my weight-training classes. I didn't know her name at that time, but she was a regular of my 3-day-a-week Turbo Kick workouts. She had been coming for years to the cardio workouts, so it was a pleasant surprise to see her up at the crack of dawn (5:30 a.m.) joining me for a strength-training workout.

"I want to get lean," she told me.

"Oh yeah?" I replied.

"I just don't want to be old and fat anymore, and I know this girl who lost 50 percent of her body fat when she started doing your weight-training classes. That's my new goal!"

I commended her on recognizing that what she had been doing wasn't working and committing to taking a new approach. Next, I explained how critical it was that she had a goal, but how refining it into a SMART goal would be more rewarding and help her achieve quicker results.

Losing 50 percent of body fat is a fantastic goal and something she would be able to achieve and maintain. But in order to reach 50 percent, we'd need to start with something SMARTer.

Getting SMART

SMART goals should be goals that can be accomplished in a realistic time frame. Most of us love instant gratification but realize that amazing results take patience. But amazing results also require momentum and motivation to stay the course. SMART health goals fuel exciting progress!

After getting a sense of what she was doing, the time she could commit to a weekly exercise program (which we determined to be about 6 hours a week), current level of determination, work schedule, family life, support of her partner, and personal willingness to learn more about nutrition and what her body needed, we were able to set a realistic and exciting short-term goal. Instead of focusing on 50 percent of her body fat, she set a SMART goal to lose 12 percent of her current body fat in 1 month's time.

Once we honed in on the foreseeable future, I could see a newfound determination in her eyes. This was doable, and in less than 4 weeks time, she'd be well on her way to achieving her overall goal of 50 percent. Since that time, Maedie has lost well in excess of 50 percent of her body fat. She looks 10 years younger. At age 52, she lifts more weight than 95 percent of my students. She's ripped. This woman went from 50, fat, and "been doing that" . . . to total hotness.

You've gone through the assignments asked of you in the first couple of days. You've set specific health and fitness goals for yourself that are a challenge but that you can achieve. However, focusing on the "end result," an ultimate number on the scale, or a specific long-term activity might not provide the mojo you need!

You can achieve all your health and fitness goals much more quickly when they are reasonable and aligned with your priorities. Your chances for success are dramatically improved by learning the best practices in setting and mastering SMART health and fitness goals.

Baby Steps and Bite-Size Pieces

The SMART goal formula I outline below will help you to generate energy, drive, enthusiasm, and amazing results with regard to your health and fitness goals. Use the SMART approach by starting with the smallest, measurable, achievable, rewarding, and time-sensitive goal on your list.

SMALLEST

Yesterday we decided which of your life goals you should tackle first: your Push goal. Now let's turn to your health and fitness goal. Unlike life goals, when it comes to our health and fitness, our primary objective is to create momentum. Following through on the smallest of objectives can create momentum. So pick a health and fitness goal that with determination and reasonable expectations you're confident you can achieve in a time frame of 2 to 4 weeks. Start there. If when you review your health and fitness goals you find most all of them require more time to accomplish, no problem! Just pick the one that's most exciting and let's chop it up!

Take a look at the goal that you isolated on Day 2. Let's say, for example, one of the most exciting goals you have listed for yourself is to run a marathon this year. Break that feat down into something you know you can knock out in less than a month. Your SMART goal might be to improve your endurance and training regimen so that in less than a month you will run/walk 3 days a week for 40 minutes. Again, it needs to be an achievement that will excite you to have accomplished in less than a month's time, something you'll feel great about and something that will motivate you to move forward. Take a moment to glance at your list and see what you can reconfigure into smaller pieces. Think "bite-size."

MEASURABLE

Review the health and fitness goal (or goals) you set for yourself on Day 2. Take the time to make sure that each health or fitness goal you've set has a "measure." A great way to describe measure is to say that an outsider would be able to evaluate whether or not you achieved your goal, beyond simply taking your word for it. For example, to set an objective to feel better is a wonderful goal, but it lacks any real means by which to know if you've achieved it. Make your goals measurable. Whatever your goal, a good place to start is with a numerical value to assess progress. Fitness goals could be the number of days per week you want to exercise. A weight-loss goal might include the number of pounds you want to lose in 30 days. Health goals could include reducing your blood pressure to a certain number or the average number of hours you plan to sleep each night. For Maedie, it meant beginning her 4-week journey by having her body fat tested. Knowing her starting mark would allow her to accurately measure her progress. With a goal of a 12 percent overall body-fat loss in 1 month, she had a clear measurement and a big red bull's-eye to aim for.

ACHIEVABLE

There's a big difference between "possible" goals and those that are realistic and "achievable." If you've ever known a wrestler who has to cut weight for a weekend tournament, you know it's possible to starve yourself, live in one of those plastic body suits, take water pills, and overexercise to drop as much as 18 pounds in a week. But I think we can all agree that's a train wreck waiting to happen.

Know the difference between the achievable and possible but simply unrealistic. A person with bad knees and disdain for running is not likely to attain her goal to win her division in the Boston Marathon this year. Goals must push you, but they must be attainable, healthy, and aligned with your priorities. Set yourself up for success by beginning with the smallest, most achievable goal on your list. Enhance the likelihood of your goals by beginning with the health and fitness goal that has the least possible obstacles. For Maedie, her initial goal was to reduce her total body fat by 50 percent. She likely would have found herself discouraged and disappointed 2 months later when she had not yet hit her mark. Losing 50 percent of your body fat in 8 weeks' time *is* possible but very unrealistic and likely unsafe. So rather than simply ask if your SMART goal can be achieved in 2 to 4 weeks, go one step further and ask yourself if it's realistic, safe, and consistent with your priorities. To aim toward her SMART goal, Maedie added 1 extra hour of working-out time, which was consistent with her lifestyle, her priorities, and long-term maintainable results.

REWARDING

You'll need to exercise a degree of willpower and make sacrifices in pursuit of your goals, and the bigger the goal, the more rewarding the achievement. But to begin, I want you to identify a smaller goal, with measurement, that you know is achievable. Identify any positive side effect of accomplishing this goal. List all the benefits and rewards, no matter how small, associated with hitting your mark! For example, if your health and fitness goal is to have a serving of vegetables at every meal, you might list the following as rewards: improved energy, feel better about myself, reduce my intake of processed and junk food, receive the nutrients my body needs to get through my workouts, improved digestion, reduced calorie intake, and decreased sugar cravings. It goes without saying that every time you check one of your goals off your list, you'll feel a surge of confidence and momentum.

TIME SENSITIVE

Each of your goals should have a measure *and* a time-specific deadline. When you set a date to achieve your goal, you give yourself a deadline. When we have deadlines, we automatically work toward those pending deadlines as our top priorities. We become more focused. Working toward a goal without a definite deadline will diminish your commitment. Nothing keeps you accountable like the calendar! For Maedie, knowing that at the end of the month she had a scheduled body-fat testing with plenty of people rooting for her, the time sensitivity of her SMART goal created powerful accountability. Select the smallest goal, with measurement, that you know you can achieve by a certain date!

Now What?

You're about to get your homework for the day. I suspect that your SMART goal will be achieved before the end of the week. So then what? Your next step after achieving your first SMART goal is simply to keep selecting the SMART goal from those that remain! You'll blow through all 10 before you know it! However, don't be shy about adding more than 10 goals! Why not? This is the year you push to be the person you know you have the potential to be. Keep the SMART formula in mind to build the bangin' body you want!

1. Refer to the goal worksheet from Day 2 and identify which of the 10 goals is your SMART (Smallest, Measurable, Achievable, Rewarding, and Time Sensitive) health and fitness goal.

2. Write your SMART goal across the top of the health and fitness goal worksheet, print, and post!

3. Create a list of all the positive side effects of achieving this first goal.

NOTES

_____

_____

_____

_____

_____

_____

_____

_____

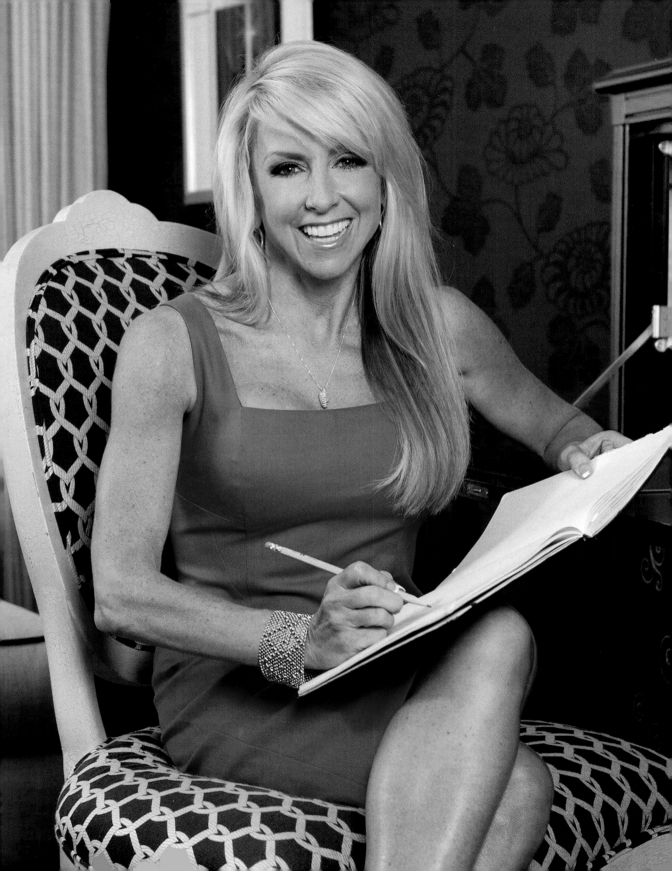

Reverse Engineering Your PUSH GOAL

Mapping Your Course

The goals worksheet got you really thinking! You're superexcited about not just mastering your health but also accomplishing some really big things this year. Are the 10 goals on your goals worksheet worth another 5 minutes? Good! Today I'm going to teach you how to "reverse engineer" your goals.

To reverse engineer something is to take it apart and figure out its inner workings before you begin to build your own version. I'm going to show you exactly how to do this. Why? All too often, we allow inertia or sheer excitement to drive our direction. But if you want to get somewhere in particular, start with a goal (and remember that all goals have been accomplished by someone else before you). Take it apart. Rip out the seams. Study how it was crafted and the labor that went into its construction. Then reduce it to specific action steps. While it can be an arduous process, when you reverse engineer a goal, you map your course to success. You create a step-by-step roadmap on your terms.

At the beginning of this book, I shared my

intention to prove beyond a shadow of a doubt that your health and fitness do not exist independently of the other areas of your life. Every facet of who you are and what you do is interrelated to the other parts. The balance and achievement you can create in one area overlap and impact the success of your overall health and fitness. I know that to be true. To create a "diet book" and not teach you what I know to be true would be wrong. No thanks, that's not how I work.

Sure, I could teach you how to reverse engineer your health and fitness goal (which is tomorrow's assignment) and hope that you understand how that would apply to your Push goal. But why not reverse engineer both? How cool would it be if you were fit and healthy *and* were able to reach your outrageously cool financial goals this year? Can I get a *woot woot!* Thank you.

Today you'll learn to create actionable steps that will bring your goals to fruition faster than you ever imagined. You will also learn the importance of flexibility and the critical skill of recognizing if and when a goal may not align with your top priorities.

Put It in Reverse— And Floor It!

Many well-meaning goals end up in the landfill of unfulfilled dreams simply because few know and execute the art of reverse engineering a goal. I want to share a personal story of how I recently reverse engineered a goal. (This is Part 1 of the tale . . . see page 39 for Part 2!)

In 2010, Bret and I took the kids on a snowboarding trip to Park City, Utah. It was New Year's Day, so naturally as we rode up the gondola, Bret and I were in goal-setting mode. Lifelong skiers, we had decided to try something new a few years back and took snowboarding lessons. (*Marriage tip:* When you have an opportunity to work to develop new hobbies together as a family or couple, take it!)

One lesson and we were hooked. We sucked at first and spent a lot of time on our butts, but as we laughed (and mocked each other), we could tell this was going to be cool. (Later, in Day 11, when I explain how to find your "soul-mate workout," you'll understand how I used my soul-mate workout formula to identify snowboarding as something that would fulfill our "feel good" exercise quotients.)

Soon we had the kids learning to "ride" with us. The decision to do something outside of our comfort zone and take that first snowboarding lesson has brought our family closer together than any other I can think of. It's a rush of adrenaline, pride, and pure joy to fly down a freshly dusted mountain at top speeds with my son, daughter, and husband shredding powder all around me! It's amazing! I can't think of many sporting activities that the whole family can enjoy together for hours on end.

The physicality of the sport is exhilarating. I love the fashion, and I love creating my own playlists and having something that pushes me to improve or be left behind! In fact, the kids tease me that my snowboarding fashion sense is better than my actual skill. I'll take that.

We've come to be passionate about snowboarding. We love what it's done for our family

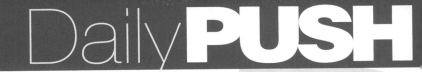

Today's Homework

BRAINSTORM YOUR PUSH GOAL

Your assignment for today is simply to create a master brainstorm for your Push goal. I have provided a sheet for you here, but in the interest of saving trees, it's only one page and I've already explained to you that I want your brainstorm to be several pages long. Be my guest in creating your master brainstorm in a journal or on a legal pad.

My Push Goal: _____

My Master Brainstorm List: _____

_____

_____

_____

_____

_____

_____

_____

_____

_____

_____

_____

and athletic pursuits so much that we've all but forced our friends to take up the sport. We realize it's become a serious obsession for us! Lightbulb!

Three Simple Steps to Success

So as we rode to the top of the mountain that snowy January 1, we decided to take our passion (as we have before) and start a new branch of our business. We declared that our 2010 Push goal was to launch a women's snowboarding apparel company. In fact, on the flight home, with a legal pad between us, we began the brain dump that is the first step of reverse engineering any big goal.

STEP ONE With pen to paper, create a master "brain dump." This is the process of brainstorming absolutely everything and anything you're going to need to know, do, acquire, master, and so on to achieve your goal.

The brain dump Bret and I created ended up being about three full pages of scribbles. I'll save you the ugly details, but here's a glimpse into the randomness of what a brainstorm should look like:

- Research spending habits of 30- to 45-year-old female snowboarders.

- Find out how many 30- to 45-year-old women currently snowboard on an annual basis.

- What is the growth rate of this segment of the population?

- Search availability of new domain name.

- Call _____ for a meeting about the business.

- Research who our competitors are using for manufacturing.

- Research industry trade show event—date and location.

- Register for trade show event.

- Research average markup, profit margin on outerwear.

The beauty of a brainstorm is that it doesn't matter in what order the information comes to you. From creating a logo to researching start-up costs, ordering letterhead, and doing a preliminary Google search on your competition, no item is too small. As a matter of fact, the further you can break down each individual action, the better.

By the way . . . notice how the word *research* keeps popping up? Research—knowing what you don't know, and knowing how to find out—is a critical part of step one. Keep reading to find out how critical.

STEP TWO Every task you write down should take 1 day, max, to complete. Break down large tasks into smaller components. For example, instead of the blanket statement "organize the garage," devise a list of smaller steps—say, buy plastic storage bins, schedule times for donation pickup, buy cleaning supplies, set a budget for garage makeover (don't forget new shelving, storage bins, tool rack, bike rack, etc.), create a sketch of what you want the garage to look like, talk to spouse about what things she/he needs access to daily, Google search "how to organize your garage," and so on.

That snippet you just read of my and Bret's brainstorming list? The complete list was very long, yet it took only about 20 minutes to create. Believe it or not, a long list is a good sign. It means that you've broken down goals into smaller and smaller pieces. A long list will help you break plateaus and the dreaded "now what?" question that so often becomes an obstacle.

STEP THREE Create a realistic schedule of how long each task should take and the proposed completion/execution day. If, like most people, you simply pick a day to end the experiment in hoarding that's going on in your garage, 8 hours later you'd probably find yourself dirty, frustrated, and halfway through the mess. Maybe you'd reward yourself with a monster-size meal and resolve to finish the garage project next weekend. I think we both know how that story ends.

When you reverse engineer goals, you quickly learn how even the most awe-inspiring challenge can be sliced into easy-to-swallow bits. You're probably nodding and saying, "Yeah, yeah, I know that already." I'm sure you do. But few people actually do it, and I know even fewer who have learned to do it effectively with their health goals.

These three steps can save you hours and help you create a simple plan that keeps you motivated, organized, and focused on the end result. With the right planning, you learn how to maintain an organized garage forever, like that guy four doors down.

Do Your Research! A Cautionary Tale

No matter how awesome your goal is, don't rush in without fully understanding how pursuing and achieving it will impact your lifestyle and your commitment to your top priority. Research is the only way to gain this understanding.

Whether you're brainstorming a Push goal or a health goal, your initial research should answer these questions:

"Why do I want to do this in the first place?"

"Does this fit with my priorities?"

The Smartphone Advantage

Create your master brainstorm on your smartphone. It's digital, so you can copy, paste, and move items around. And unlike a paper list, your smartphone list will always be at hand. You'll never have to wonder where you put it.

Another great reason to keep your master brainstorm on your phone: I suspect that, just when you *think* you've exhausted your list, some really great ideas may come to you. Not to worry. Your phone is right there. Just add your new thoughts!

"What is really involved?"

"What is my very first step?"

There's a very good reason to ponder these questions. Thank God Bret and I did.

As part of our research, Bret and I needed to find out if owning and operating a snowboarding company fit with our top priority clarity statement. (Remember this? If not, flip back to Day 1.) So we scheduled a meeting with our friend Andy, who had owned and operated a similar business.

In the first 10 minutes of our lunch meeting, Andy asked a few questions. The first two gave

Daily**PUSH**

There's only one item to add to your to-do list today. One, because this one needs your full attention!

1. Master brainstorm: List everything and anything that relates to accomplishing your PUSH goal. This list should range from small (a Google search) to big (a business plan). Don't worry about how this list is ordered. Just write down everything you might need to know, learn, do, think, find, research, sketch, or understand as it relates to your PUSH goal.

NOTES

_____

_____

_____

_____

_____

_____

_____

_____

us pause: "Are you ready to turn your hobby and your fun escape into a full-time job?" and "Are you prepared to spend the majority of your vacation visiting accounts, making appearances, and servicing your customers?"

But his *third* question was a killer: "Are you ready to work really hard to learn everything you need to know about a business you know nothing about—without the help of celebrity contacts—and that is notoriously hard to turn a profit in?"

Sccrrreeeeeeeech! That's the sound of us slamming on the brakes when we realized none of the above fit with our priorities or already balanced lifestyle. Duh! What were we thinking?!?

But hey, no worries. Because we'd made a list of 10 goals for 2010, we were able to quickly move to the next goal that we assessed to be our Push goal. So out with snowboard gear and in with next Push goal: helping 100,000 people by creating a free online video coaching program on organizing your life. Just a few days into our research for that goal, we realized everything about it fit with our top priority clarity statement. It really was a better fit for my second and third priorities.

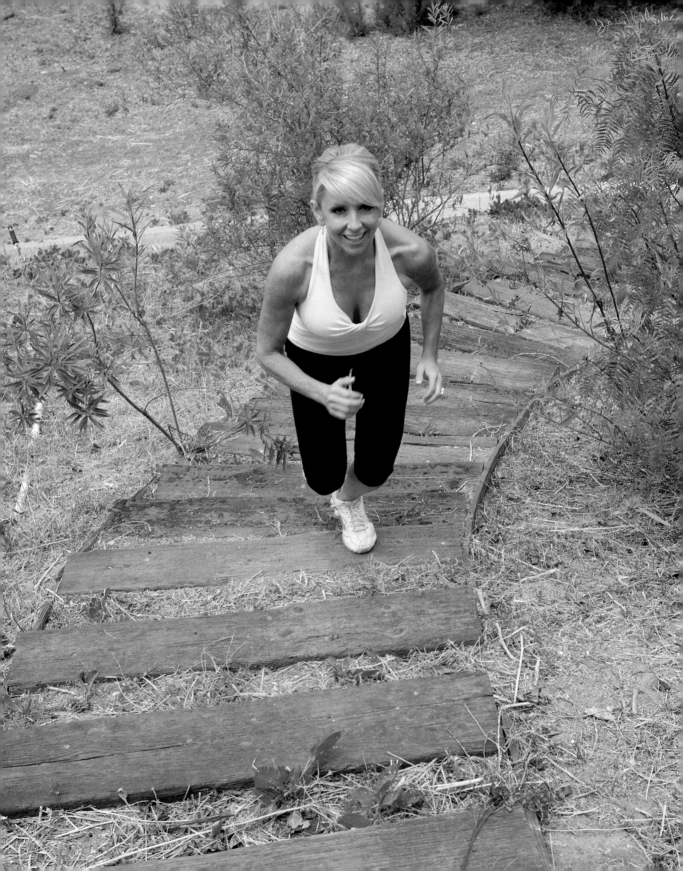

Reverse Engineering Your HEALTH GOAL

How to Get from Here to the Hot Body You Deserve

As you know from Day 5, to reverse engineer something is to take it apart and study how it was put together. As a kid, I was fascinated by telephones. Remember the old rotary phones with the curly cords? They're probably collectors' items now. I bet I'm not the only one who unscrewed the ear- and mouthpieces to have a look inside. I'd guess the guy who built your house actually took the whole phone apart.

As I was leaving the gym recently, one of my students stopped me to ask if I thought her goal to lose 30 pounds in 2 months was realistic. I asked her how many pounds per week she was comfortable trying to lose. "I really haven't bro- ken it down that way yet," she admitted. Then I asked, "How many calories are you burning on average right now, and do you know what your body fat is?" Again she replied, "Well, I need to figure that out." I followed that with, "Well, how hard are you willing to work?" She smirked at me, as if to take the hint, and said, "I guess what you're saying is I need to do a little research first, huh?"

Reverse engineering is common practice in business and finance. Yet when it comes to your health goal, it is equally important! My student's goal to lose 30 pounds in 2 months might be very doable, or a 3-month time frame might be more realistic based on her individual situation. There's only one way to know, and that is to figure out what it would take to get there—deconstruct the goal!

Anything you seek to accomplish in the next 12 months, someone has done it before you. That's great news! It means you too can accomplish the same feat. It also means the blow-by-blow steps you need to get where you're going have already been mapped for you. In the words of my friend Brian Tracy, "No one is smarter than you. And no one is better than you." In other words, you can do anything you set your mind to. If someone else has lost 100 pounds or gotten himself out of debt, so can you, but you need the blueprint.

Grab a flathead screwdriver, some duct tape, and a hammer. Before we start out in the direction of a brand-new you, we'll need to map our course. Today we're going to disassemble your health goal. We're going to figure out where you want to be and work backward to determine exactly what it will take to get there.

Before we begin, here's a reminder: Your health goal needs a relatively precise measure. To list "Have more energy" is fan-tab-ulous, but we need a way specifically to measure it. No sissy goals. Put it out there. Believe! Set your sights high! Make sure your health goal includes quantifications such as a number, a measurement, a body-fat percentage, a number of miles you can run, a number of days you will exercise each week, etc. Measurements give you direction and hold you accountable.

Reverse Your Way to Health

Let's say your health goal is to lose 20 pounds and cut your body fat in half. You can picture yourself at your birthday celebration next year in a great new outfit and looking toned and sexy. A list that simply states "lose 20 pounds, exercise more, eat less, and join a gym" is like walking into the forest without a map and compass.

Instead, I want you to create a brainstorm list of everything you could possible need to know, do, change, research, buy, organize, and schedule to make this goal happen. Essentially, you're repeating the exercise of Day 5, but specifically for your health.

I've given you a sample brainstorming list below. It's long, but long lists are good. In fact, long lists are superior! Each line of your brainstorm represents a small step, a detailed guide. Make your list as long as possible. (P.S. I'll answer many of the questions below in subsequent pages! So start your research with this book!)

- How much weight do I want to lose per week?

- How much of a calorie deficit would I need to create to lose 2 pounds per week?

- How many calories per day does my body burn right now?

- Based on my estimated current calorie burn, how many calories per day I should consume?

- Have my body fat measured:
  - Research cost of hydrostatic body-fat testing in my area.
  - Have a reputable personal trainer measure my body fat.

- What should my body-fat percentage be?

- Find an online support forum for fitness people.

- From the message boards, interview someone who was able to reduce her body fat by 50 percent.

- Create a very detailed list of questions for this person.

- Interview a second person. (Find someone who started where I am now.)

- Research what a reasonable length of time it takes to reduce body fat by 50 percent.

- Research which exercise routines help reduce body fat the most effectively.

- Complete the soul-mate workout worksheet (see Day 11, page 78).

- Set two dates this week to sample new workouts.

- Look into the cost of gym membership.

- Research the cost of equipment I might need. (Purchase used?)

- Rearrange my schedule to allow for early a.m. workout.

- Budget to buy a calorie-counting device.

- Buy portable containers suggested by Chalene.

- Find an online accountability partner.

- Sell my old laptop and use the money for new cross trainers.

- Take before photos on my cell phone (for my eyes only).

- Organize the pantry.

- Organize the fridge.

- Throw out all the junk.

- Put an alert in my phone to remind me to eat every 3 hours.

- Put an alert on my phone that reminds me to review my Push and health goals.

- Pull the smaller dinner plates from storage.

- Schedule a date for weekly progress photos.

- Make a promise to my accountability partner to send him or her my pics.

- Subscribe to two free nutrition newsletters.

- Use my phone to snap pics of everything I eat all day for accountability/accuracy.

- Find an expert in vegan cooking.

- Schedule all workouts for this week.

- Learn everything I can about exercising with a knee injury.

- Start a lunchtime walking program at work.

- Ask my family and co-workers for their support.

- Ask my family and co-workers to join me on my quest to be healthy for life! (Remember, this is my new lifestyle!)

- Schedule times on my calendar for meal prep for the week on Sundays/Wednesdays.

- Talk to a few people about their "diet."

- Research the best fine dining options for healthy folks and what/how to order.

- Research the best app for calorie tracking.

- Look at free Web sites that help me determine my daily calorie burn.

- Track my calories daily using my phone.

- Organize my food prep area to have measuring cups, scale, etc., easily accessible.

- Make a list of the negative things I say to myself and replace them with the opposite.

- Sign up for free accountability coaching at one of the Web sites listed by Chalene.

- Schedule a physical with my doc.

- Talk the girls into changing bunco/wine night into a power walk Saturday.

- Keep a journal of how I feel after I exercise.

- Post a list of all the adjectives I will feel when I'm healthy for life—post it on the fridge.

- Create a list of favorite activities other than my soul-mate workout.

- Make a promise to my husband and my co-workers that I will be losing 20 pounds by x date and that it will be gone for good!

- Get a water purifier.

- Dust off my George Foreman grill.

- Grocery shop with a list.

- Keep myself accountable with a video diary and post it to my blog.

- Schedule a weigh-in date with my accountability partner.

- Schedule a monthly follow-up body-fat testing—post results to my blog.

- Decide what foods I need to just stop buying.

- Ask friends for suggestions on their favorite workout DVDs.

- Create a playlist of the songs that pump me up!

- Cancel my rag mags and replace with health subscriptions.

- Schedule a weekly family walk on Sunday.

- Keep a gratitude journal.

- Volunteer to help with PE at the kids' school.

- Call my neighbor and see if she wants to do this with me.

Your assignment for today is to create a master brainstorm for your health goal, just as you did for your Push goal. I have provided a sheet for you here, but in the interest of saving trees, it's only one page, and I've already explained that I want your brainstorm to be several pages long! Be my guest in creating your master brainstorm in a journal or on a legal pad.

My Push Goal: _____

My Master Brainstorm List: _____

_____

_____

_____

_____

_____

_____

_____

_____

_____

_____

_____

_____

_____

_____

SUCCESS
Is Your
ONLY OPTION

You're the Head Coach for Team YOU

Fun! Fun! Fun! You'll like this. Today we customize your definition of success.

I'll go first. I have learned enough about what makes me feel happy and successful to know that it boils down to just one word . . . *choice.*

I asked some of my online friends to share their definition of success.

Jane Greene Success is when you're falling asleep with a smile and excited for the next day's challenge.

Pam Jones Success is being secure enough in yourself and your surroundings to be yourself and flourish in all you do!

Layla Mitchell When you can wake up in the morning and KNOW that you are happy with where you are and what you have . . . then you've succeeded.

Brett Hammond Success is many different things to me. To be the most successful, I want to be happy, have the freedom to do whatever my heart desires, and have a sense of accomplishment as I check things off my to-do list.

Kim Solomon Success to me is living life without obligation, but with purpose and passion.

And perhaps my favorite:

Katrina Ferris Success is that inner feeling of PEACE when you know you have given it 100% and you have made a difference, even if it's just in one person's life. It's not about money, power, fame, or just yourself. It's about surrounding yourself with positive people and moving forward, only to look back to learn from your mistakes. It's about falling flat on your face and showing others that it is okay to fail and you can get back up. It's showing others that it's not a weakness to take hold of that hand reaching out to you for assistance and guidance. Success is PAYING it forward everyday; we ARE all connected.

For success to be your only option, you must create a definition that grabs you by the heartstrings. Your personal definition of success must motivate you in such a way that you will do whatever it takes to achieve it.

"The Only Option" Attitude

When you believe all the way to your bones that success is your only option, you take every step possible to ensure that failure is not a possibility. Guaranteeing yourself success will take many layers of accountability and foster in you the resolve that every obstacle you encounter can and must be overcome. You will find a way.

Your success is 100 percent your responsibility, and yours alone. There's no room for excuses. There is no point in blaming your spouse, your parents, your financial situation, the color of your hair . . . whatever. Many others in far worse situations than your own have succeeded at accomplishing the very same goals you have set for yourself. Excuses are for the weak. Success is your only option and you *will* take the steps necessary to ensure it!

The first person you'll need to find is a great coach!

Congratulations! You're Hired!

Grab a clipboard, some tight polyester shorts, and a whistle. You've just been appointed the head coach of the most important team on the planet: yours. You are the person who will coach your team of one to success.

And you need to be a damn good coach, too! So start working on it! You'll need to stop yourself from using anything but positive, performance-inspiring phrases.

When meeting their fiercest opponents, great coaches deliver fire-filled, awe-inspiring pregame speeches. Their words inspire the smallest player to run right through the biggest opponent. They don't speak of physical brawn or past defeats; they speak to the heart of the player. The heart of a winner believes that success is the only option.

Can you be that coach?

Learning to Be a Great Coach

Can you imagine a coach sitting down with his team and saying, "Hey, guys, I don't know if you can do this. I've seen what you're up against out there, and it doesn't look good. Plus, we're pretty small. We don't have the right equipment, and our field isn't as nice as the one they practice on." That team would lose.

The voice you hear in your head that makes you doubt yourself is the voice that repeats negative phrases. You might think of it as just venting to yourself, but your words pack power.

To be a great coach, you have to believe in the heart of your team. Size and circumstance are irrelevant. You must put an end to self-limiting phrases. Statements like "I can't handle this," "I can't do this," "I will always be fat," "I'm under

Daily PUSH

1. Write out your own definition of success.

2. Add action items to your to-do list that specifically address your environment of success. Examples: "Schedule 2 hours to declutter my desk" and "Set up a special area in the garage for my workouts."

NOTES

_____

_____

_____

_____

_____

_____

_____

_____

too much stress," "I'm not good enough," and "I know I'll fail" will guarantee derailment.

The words you speak can serve you or hurt you. The cruelest words you've ever heard were probably in your own head. Would you speak with such cruelty to a child or to anyone you wanted to succeed? Of course not! The words you use to describe yourself, whether in your own head or spoken to others, can either unleash or limit your own potential. You have a choice. The words you use are habitual. Speaking to yourself like a legendary winning coach is a skill and a habit you can develop.

You're going to flip the switch on right now. From this moment forward, you will eliminate the habit of speaking to yourself negatively. Yup, you're going cold turkey on this one!

So coach yourself like you *must* win. Resolve to do the things you find to be difficult. That's what confident people do. They tackle those things that are scary and they get addicted to doing it. They set a new goal and they tackle it. They do what others will not, and that gives them confidence. To have confidence is to know that your challenges are not going to kill you. You can do it. You might not be great at it at first, but eventually you'll get it down. And the more you do it, the better you'll become.

Visualize Your Success

Think of yourself as if you were already that successful person you want to be. Instead of saying "I'm fat and out of shape," replace those phrases with what it is you desire: "I'm strong. I'm getting leaner. I'm a fighter. I'm starting this journey and I'm going to complete it." The key is habitually thinking of yourself as the success that you are becoming.

Success in any area isn't something that just happens. Becoming successful mandates change. You must learn the habits that will ensure your success. Each of your goals will be achieved because you are committed to forming the habits required and building the foundation that it takes to succeed.

You're 7 days in.

Success is your only option.

Create an Environment to Succeed

Some of your worst habits arise from being in a negative or unhealthy environment. "Environment" includes the physical space that you spend the most time in as well as the people with whom you spend your time. Does your environment make your success more attainable or more difficult? Create the environment you need to support your mission.

I don't know which came first, the chicken or the egg. But about the time that I learned to create a special type of to-do list, every part of my environment started to become more organized. As I organized my priorities and set goals, my car got more organized. As the habit of checking my to-do list several times a day solidified, my closet seemed to get neater. As I began to think with clarity, my environment became decluttered.

The same is happening for you. It's not by chance—it is purposeful.

DAY 8

MAPPING
Your Course

The Game Plan for Reaching Your Goals

This is crazy. Can you taste it? You're so close! I know we're only 8 days in, but you have made it to a place on the road to success that most people never see. By this time, most people have already flipped ahead for a shortcut and lost their way. Not you. Not this time. (Have I mentioned that *PUSH* is so much bigger than a diet?)

The momentum from the few steps I'll walk you through today will propel you in the direction of your goals with an energy and speed you've never experienced before.

On Days 5 and 6, you reverse engineered your Push and health goals. You created a massive brainstorm, a list of actions. Now we'll organize that list into a plan, and just minutes from now you'll be on your course!

It took some work to get to this day. It wasn't rocket science, but it did require disciplining yourself to slow down, sit down, and write down what you wanted for yourself.

But here's the big question: What exactly do you do next? Today you find out!

How to Get Where You Want to Go

There are bazillions of books, articles, and Web sites devoted to goal setting and achievement. I've read half of them. But I still haven't found one that walks you through those first steps.

Define priorities. *Check.* Set goals. *Check.* Reverse engineer. *Check.* But then what? What am I supposed to do tomorrow and the next day? What's first? What if I make a mistake? How do I get to where I've decided I want to go? That's what most goal-achievement programs never cover.

Fifteen years ago, when I set out to understand goal setting and learn how to reverse engineer my desires, I remember getting to this exact point, the point where you are today. Being at this stage is like setting out to prepare a four-course meal for the first time. You've just returned from the market with three bags of the finest ingredients. With your own taste in mind, you've selected the most delicious of entrees. You're home from the market and you've displayed each ingredient on the counter. You're ready to get started . . . only you have no idea what to do first. Now what?

All those expensive ingredients laid out in front of you can be a bit overwhelming. Not to fear! You're about to learn how to create cooking instructions from your reverse-engineered brainstorm. Even better news: By the end of today's lesson, you'll be able to create step-by-step cooking instructions for any goal, for every goal!

The work that you've done to reverse engineer your Push and health goals now provides the vital ingredients you need to plan for tomorrow, the next day, next week, and the next 20 days.

First Steps

When I interview people who have successfully turned their lives around physically, professionally, or spiritually, I always ask, "What advice would the *new* you give the *old* you?" They always respond vehemently, "Just start!"

Start today. For some people, those first couple of steps are challenging because they find themselves so concerned that they might do things in the wrong order. Congratulations! You're already waaaaaay past that hurdle. Your master brainstorm is your fast-pass! You've already created an exhaustive list to get you from here to *there.* All movement creates momentum. All momentum is progress. So don't worry too much about the exact order of things. As a rule, however, always start with tasks that relate to research and information gathering.

Research is what helps you make an informed decision on whether a goal is right for you before you invest too much time, energy, and resources pursuing it. You have to be flexible about the goals you listed on your worksheet. If and when you find yourself in a position where your research suggests that a particular goal doesn't fit with your priorities (as Bret and I did with our quest to start a snowboarding apparel company), then you cross that one off the list and come up with a new goal to fill its spot.

You're going to have 10 really amazing things happen for you this year; don't shortchange yourself.

As an example, let's use the plan to start a snowboarding apparel company. Looking at the reverse-engineering brainstorm list on page 34, we want to start with research, but while we're learning more about your goal, we also need to get moving in that direction.

Once again, get a pen and paper. You'll also need your reverse-engineered brainstorm list. It's up to you which you'd like to do first, as you will eventually do both! (Pushy . . . *I know*.)

Create four columns on your page. Write these four headings at the top of the columns.

RESEARCH   FIRST   DURING   LATER

Here's the long definition for each category:

RESEARCH List in this column any task that relates to learning more about whether your goal is right for you. That includes learning what you need to know about what it will take and interviewing or studying those who have done it before you. Your first action steps will be centered around research that will help you answer the following question: "Does this make sense for me? Am I willing to do the work?"

FIRST Items that go in this column are those things you'll do first *after* your research confirms the appropriateness of your goal. That is, you've decided that, based on solid knowledge, your goal makes sense, that the work and circumstances involved do not conflict with your priorities. This column should also begin with additional research that will help you become an expert and make informed decisions. As you exhaust your list of things to to research, you'll begin adding action steps to this column as well. Research tasks that could go in this column might include "research local snowboarding apparel manufacturers," "research trademark expenses," or "research trademark availability."

Beginning action steps in this column might include "fill out online trademark registration" and "schedule meeting with Lisa the pattern-maker."

DURING These are action items that you must be doing along the way. Say, for example, you're mapping out the course of your health goal. On your "During" list would be "exercise every day" and "Track my daily calorie burn and calorie intake."

When I created this list for my goal of speaking with Brian Tracy, regardless of the stage at which I was in the process, I also needed to be working on my speaking and networking skills. If Bret and I had decided to move forward with our idea to start a snowboarding apparel company, throughout the entire process we would have needed to be working on building a list of clients. It wouldn't make any sense to spend 12 months building a great apparel company, accept delivery of thousands of dollars' worth of apparel, and then to not have put 12 months' worth of effort into establishing a fan base or retailers to buy our product.

My best friend Monica Gray loves to tell people about the children's T-shirt company she started. Her reverse-engineered brainstorm included all the first steps, all the later steps, but it was the missing the During steps. When hundreds boxes of garments were ready for pickup, she had a place to store them but nowhere to sell them. She had spent thousands of dollars and hundreds of hours planning her business, creating a darling product line, but she missed a step. She omitted the activities that needed to be addressed "during" the journey to goal achievements. Now she would have to spend the next 12 months building a customer list, working to establish her line with children's boutiques, or selling them door to door. Doing that after the product arrived meant the loss of precious time as trends in children's clothing marched onward. `LATER` Anything that doesn't have to be done in the first 30 days can go in this column. Anything that can wait, that doesn't make sense to do now, you will add to this column. So let's say that your health goal is to lose 40 pounds. Items that might be placed in the Later column could include: Look into alternative workouts other than running during the winter months, schedule a photo shoot, buy new clothes, or begin training for a marathon. While all of these action items are on your reverse-engineered brainstorm list, they're down the road.

Let me put your mind at ease. *You can't make a mistake here.* As long as you're pushing forward, you're winning! Every day that you add action items to your to-do list you are 1 day closer to goal achievement.

Go Beyond Mere Productivity

Notice that we're not using a to-do list just to remind ourselves to pick up the dry cleaning. Oh sure, errands will still make the cut, but by going the extra step of adding just two or three action items from these columns to your to-do list, you move from simply being the most organized person on the block to actually living the life you deserve.

WHERE TO STORE YOUR MAP

Each day, when you craft your daily to-do list, you will refer to these columns. Certainly, you understand how critical and how helpful these columns become. The columns you've created will become your GPS. As such, I ask that you transfer this list to a safe place for easy and regular (daily) review. Hey! I have an idea! How about your phone? Why not? It's always with you.

EXACTLY HOW MUCH TO ADD TO YOUR LIST

Your daily to-do list will include an item (or two) from your columns that relate to nutrition or food, and one item that relates to physical fitness (i.e. exercise, sleep, monitoring calorie burn, etc.). You might wonder why an fitness expert might suggest two nutritional tasks and only one that relates to exercise. Great question. Here's your honest answer. Fully 80 percent of results will come from your nutrition. Exercise accounts for only about 20 percent.

To map out the first 10 days, I need you to have three small tasks related to achieving your health goal every day. Tasks should include:

- One physical activity
- One nutritional habit
- One knowledge/skill/tools-related task

Suppose your health goal is to lose 40 pounds. Then your first 11 days might look like this:

Day 1
- Go for a 20-minute brisk walk.
- Figure out how many calories per day I should consume.
- Find a person on Facebook or message boards who was able to reduce their body fat by 50 percent.

Day 2

- Do 20 minutes of cardio (my soul mate).
- Organize my food prep area: measuring cups, scale, containers.
- Write out list of questions to ask person who lost 50 percent body fat.

Day 3

- Do 30 minutes of strength training using Chalene's bangin' body plan.
- Add to my weekly calendar a full hour two times a week for food prep.
- Add an alert to my phone to remind me to eat every 3 hours.

Day 4

- Do 20 minutes of my favorite cardio.
- Throw out all the junk food.
- Put daily alert on my phone to review my Push and health goals.

Day 5

- Do 20 minutes of cardio/20 minutes of strength training.
- Pull the smaller dinner plates from storage.
- Buy a calorie-counting device to monitor my metabolism.

Day 6

- Do 30 minutes of cardio (soul-mate workout).
- Use my phone to snap pics of everything I eat all day for accountability.
- Subscribe to two free nutrition newsletters.

Day 7

- Take a 30-minute casual walk with a family member.
- Prep healthy lunch/dinners for the next 3 days.
- Research vegan Web sites.

Day 8

- Do a 30-minute strength workout.
- Ask my family and co-workers for their support in eating healthy.
- Research the best dining options for healthy food (what/how to order).

Day 9

- Do a 33-minute nonimpact workout (recumbent bike?).
- Start recording my daily calorie intake on food journal app.
- Research the best app for calorie counting on my phone.

Day 10

- Do a 30-minute workout that I've never tried before.
- Reorganize my pantry and fridge.
- Buy a water container that fits in my car's cup holder.

Day 11

- Have body fat tested.
- Pull out my blender and grilling machine/recipes.
- Buy portable containers suggested by Chalene.

Your Push Goal

As you might expect, you'll do nearly the same thing for your Push goal, and the process is even easier! All you need to do is pluck one or two items from your "research" column. Once you've worked your way through that list, which could quite possibly take less than a week, you'll begin by taking items from your First and During lists.

Just two or three tasks per day that take less than 15 minutes, most of which can be done from your desktop, will go on your to-do list. In the next few days, you'll learn exactly how simple this to-do list stuff can be!

But before we get there, you might be dying to know what your to-do list will look like with tasks related to your Push goal, your health goal, and all the things that life throws at us on a daily basis? Not that bad! I promise. Probably something like this:

- Do a 33-minute nonimpact workout (recumbent bike?)—33 minutes

- Start recording my calorie intake daily on food journal app—3 minutes

- Research the best app for calorie counts on food to use on my phone—5 minutes

- Research online trademark registration—12 minutes

- Research patternmakers in my area on Google—6 minutes

Okay, aside from the exercise, which is really about as negotiable as regular hygiene, the remaining tasks take about 26 minutes. Do you think you could skip 26 minutes of watching TV tonight to be that much closer to the life you deserve? For Pete's sake, you could do each and every one of those tasks with the TV on in the background if you have to!

It's Time

Do you want a better life? Do you want to achieve the goals you've set for yourself, physically, spiritually, professionally, financially? If the answer is yes, then you have one choice. You must do things differently. Period.

If you *try*, it won't work. I promise you that. You must *take action*. Now.

You have more than hopes and dreams. You have a destination, and we've mapped the course. More than that, you have the tools. You have the skills you need to chart your course and create a detailed turn-by-turn map for any and every goal on your list. These first 8 days have been worth your effort. They will serve you the rest of your life. Master this process once, and you will return to it repeatedly for the rest of your life.

When I set out to turn my fitness program into something people could experience across the country, I followed the exact steps you have mastered in the first 8 days of this program. When I set a goal for to establish myself as a leading expert in personal development—not just fitness—one of my underlying goals was to speak with the personal development expert Brian Tracy, one of the most influential mentors in my life. I set the goal for myself in March 2010. I followed this very same process.

First, just as you have, I created a reverse-engineered brainstorm, and then I charted my course and added just a few small steps each day to move me closer. By January 2011, Mr. Tracy had asked me to share the stage with him at his Power of Personal Achievement seminar. How fitting! So how does a no-name speaker in an industry notoriously dominated by suits (in which it might normally take 20 years to make your mark) go from virtual obscurity to achieving a crazy cool goal like that? Simple. And now you can do the same.

Now you have a plan! Now you know what steps come first. Congratulations, you've gone the extra mile. As someone once said, the best part about going the extra mile is that there is very little traffic! Push the pedal to the metal. No one can stop you now!

Daily PUSH

1. Create your columns and then transfer each reverse-engineered brainstorm item to the column that fits best.

2. Do the same for your Push goal.

3. Transfer these lists to a digital device, preferably your smartphone or laptop.

NOTES

_____   _____

_____   _____

_____   _____

_____   _____

_____   _____

_____   _____

_____   _____

TO-DO LISTS

The Key to Success: Eat the Frog!

*"Eat a live frog every morning, and nothing worse
will happen to you the rest of the day."*

—Mark Twain

Today you'll learn to create a to-do list—but not just any "be more organized" kinda to-do list. Your mission, should you choose to accept it, is to learn my five-step formula for creating a list that will flip the switch on your whole life. You will learn to simplify and prioritize your tasks, decide what should come off your plate, and create a daily habit that will bring you success for the rest of your life.

I know my method will bring you success, because it's the reason for my own. In fact, when I'm asked for the secret to my financial, physical, personal, and professional success, as I often am, I respond: "It's my frog-eating to-do list!" But I didn't just have to learn it. I had to *create* it! And let me tell you, it took a while.

Like you, I always believed I had greatness in me. But the first 25 years of my life would not reflect said belief. Voted class clown of my 1987 graduating class, I got by with a B average in just about everything from school to dance lessons. I tried my hand at million different things. I never—and I mean *never*—focused on one skill or gave one pursuit my all. I wouldn't say I was a quitter, but there was always a moment I realized

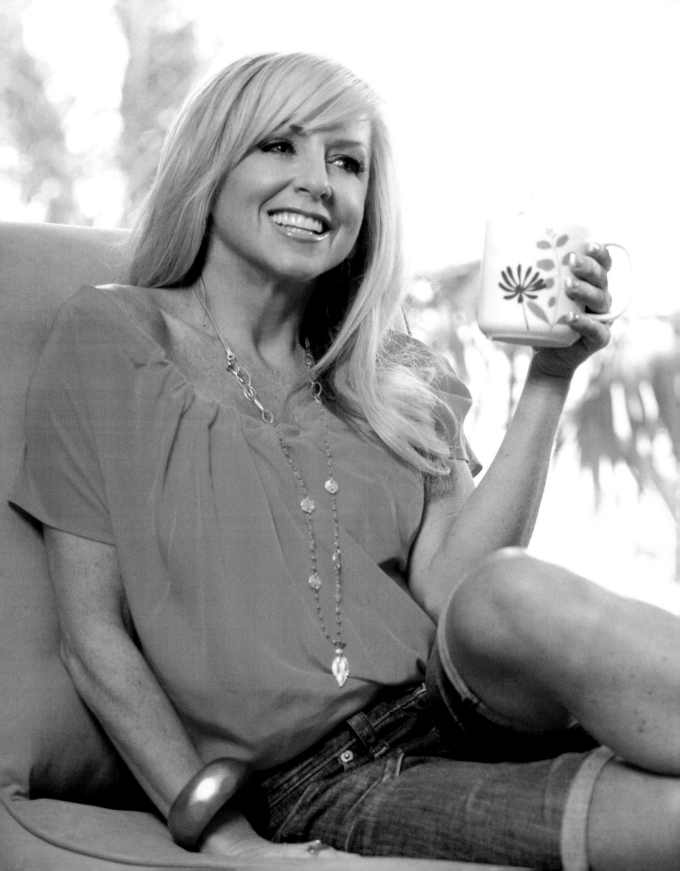

I couldn't be the best at a certain activity, whatever it was, and I didn't want to waste my time being average. In my eyes, I wasn't quitting. I was searching for my *thing*.

When I heard people talk about their life's calling, their "true passion," or their God-given talents, I assumed I just hadn't found mine yet. But as time passed, my search seemed endless. I desperately wanted to stumble upon my passion, that *thing* that would "define" me.

In the process, I just got busier. Pulled in many directions, I never felt sure if any one of my pursuits was "the thing." I was stressed and overstretched, unsure of who I really was. I often daydreamed about how it must feel to be that überhealthy fitness professional or what it must be like to find your passion.

I assumed if I just applied a stronger work ethic and tried to "do it all," eventually I would run into "it." I even tried to convince myself that

Passing On the Power: My Purpose, My Passion

Certainly, I am not the first person to teach the importance of a daily to-do list. But I *have* harnessed its power to the power of technology, with proven results. (Just ask my clients, my friends, the comments I get on my Facebook page . . . you get the idea!)

If you've ever listened to any of my audio programs, attended one of my motivational camps, or heard one of my lectures, you know I believe that creating a to-do list is our greatest equalizer. All of my employees (many of whom have gone on to start their own successful businesses), the people I train, my children, my associates, strangers on planes, and just about anyone else who will listen will tell you that I'm more passionate about this type of to-do list than anything else.

In fact, you're far more likely to hear me talking about to-do lists than you are fitness, nutrition, or business. Truth be told, it's not the 160-plus exercise DVDs I've created that make me beam with pride, it's the thousands of people who have transformed their lives by developing this one habit. To spread the word about the power of my formula . . . is my professional purpose.

From the moment I devised my frog-eating to-do list, I've not just shared it, I've *preached* it—because I have personally seen it transform lives. Let me ask you, if you thought you'd stumbled upon a formula that would make life easier for anyone willing to try it, wouldn't you be this obsessed? Exactly!

So I say, with complete confidence, that if you learn and use this very specific method every day, you have greater potential than any other time in your life to reach the top 3 percent of your industry and be in the best shape of your life.

what I was great at was being "good" at a variety of things.

Focus. That word haunted me.

When you were a kid, did your parents lecture you about focus?

"You need to focus. Sit down. Get your homework done. Focus."

"If you want to make first string, you need to go to practice. *Focus!*"

But it wasn't until I was an adult that I understood *how* to focus and how quickly I'd meet my goals once I did.

Once I developed and mastered this method, my life changed. I realized I'd never have to stress about "getting it all done" ever again. To this day, "eating the frog" has given me the peace of mind to know that anything is possible.

Daily PUSH

EAT YOUR FROG! (A COMMITMENT TO YOURSELF)

I, _____, want to have my life be more manageable, happy, healthy, and balanced. I will therefore not "try" to keep my to-do list, I will *actually do it.* I commit to keeping a frog-eating to-do list for _____ days.*

*I hope you gave me 30 days. I suppose that's a ridiculous thing to hope for—I mean, you are supersmart. After just a few days, the payoff will be obvious! Besides, after 21 days, my formula will be a habit. Thirty days just seals the deal.

Why the Typical To-Do List Doesn't Cut It

Eat your vegetables before you have dessert. Do your homework before you go out to play. Finish your chores before you watch cartoons. The "dirty work first" concept is a parent's mandate. Our parents understood that left to our own devices, not much of importance would get done.

But somewhere around the moment we realized no one else was running our lives, many of us resorted to eating dessert first. In other words, we kept ourselves busy with the easy stuff to avoid tackling the important stuff.

Creating the life and the body you want requires action. More important, it requires taking the *right* action. This is not a book about getting more done. You don't have time for more. More is not the answer. *I'm teaching you how to get the right stuff done.* Unwritten goals without some frog-eating action are little more than wishful thinking. I will show you how to scrape junk off your plate in order to have room for the truly important stuff: meeting your goals.

Mental to-do lists are not acceptable here! Sure, from time to time, they get you by. One not-so-fateful night you resolve to wake early, exercise, prep healthy meals for the day, plot out a few errands, run a couple of phone calls, and finish by hitting the hay before the 11 o'clock news. But the next morning starts just as the previous 364, with a cup of coffee and a check-in on Facebook, which leads to e-mail hell, four

unexpected errands, a forgotten deadline, and two conference calls that went way longer than scheduled. By 3:00 p.m., your day is gone and so is your belief that you'll ever have time in your crazy schedule to get to the stuff that's really important.

It's not that you're any busier than the next person. Your solution lies in learning my five-step formula for creating a Push-goal-oriented to-do list. It will make you *unstoppable*. A few weeks from today, you'll automatically, effortlessly, prioritize your tasks each day and then unleash your tackle-the-worst-first action plan! I'm excited for you!

The To-Do Tool You Absolutely Must Have

Maybe you're wondering why I'm so excited about something as everyday as a to-do list. It's because if you use this very special, quite simple formula, this actually works—effortlessly. If you are inconsistent in making lists or if you avoid creating a daily to-do list because you assume it's complicated or time consuming (most are), I'm here to tell you that this one is not. Get ready to use your smartphone to prioritize your tasks, simplify your life, and meet your goals today!

My formula is 100 times easier when you create your list on your smartphone. Can you apply its techniques to some other method—stickie notes, a written list, the scheduler on your computer? Sure. And you can keep your cash in your shoe if that makes more sense to you.

I mean, you're carrying your phone with you 24/7 anyway. Why not actually give it a purpose?!? For about $1 an app, it becomes a personal trainer, nutritionist, calorie counter, before-and-after photographer, fitness journal, nutritional diary, accountability partner, day planner, coach, task manager, mobile classroom, even your own personal chef, and so much more. Your phone can take you from the kind of person who occasionally keeps to-do lists, scattered on Post-it notes and the back of envelopes, to one of those calmly organized folks who never seems to be short on time. So don't you dare decide before we even begin that you won't consider a smartphone or that you will use the one you have just to simplify this process. You're too smart, too committed to waste time being stubborn about this. (I'm only pushy because I care!)

If you establish and diligently maintain this daily to-do list, you will improve your peace of mind, experience less stress, minimize life clutter, improve your relationships, create more wealth, boost your self-esteem, and, above all, *create* more of the most valuable commodity you need to create a balanced life: time.

Let's begin with the basic five steps.

1. Same time: Create your to-do list at the same time every day.

2. Same place: Maintain your to-do list in one location.

3. Carry your to-do list with you at all times.

4. Begin each list with three items related to your Push goal and three related to your health goal.

5. Review and revisit your list several times per day.

Using these steps and your smartphone, you'll absolutely *blast* through your master brainstorm. Your only complaint will be that you can't come up with goals to tackle fast enough!

The Smartphone Advantage

Although they're less than 2 decades old, our cell phones have already become extensions of who we are. If you're halfway to your destination and you suddenly realize you've left your phone at home, you are more likely to make a U-turn and arrive late rather than spend the night without it. Statistics vary, but most estimate conservatively that the average American checks his or her cell phone between 24 and 50 times a day for e-mails, texts, the time, apps, social media, and that very old-fashioned phone call.

Can you imagine if just once an hour when you glanced at your phone you were reminded of the goals you're working toward? Powerful!

Step One: Same Time

Just as your exercise must become a routine and predictable part of your day (we'll get to that in Day 13), so must the time that you create your daily to-do list.

One of the easiest ways to create a habit is to make it a natural part of your routine. Feeding your pets in the a.m. or reading the morning paper are *habits* spurred by the time of the day you do them. They become rituals. When you make your list at the same time each day, the habit becomes as ingrained and entrenched as brushing your teeth when you wake up. You don't have to remind yourself, you just do it. In fact, you have only one decision to make: Should you make your to-do list first thing in the morning or should it be one of the last things you do before you go to sleep at night?

Remember that the time you select should be a time where you have total solitude. Your list should be made in an environment without distraction. No noise. No one needs your attention. The TV isn't playing in the background. You aren't responding to phone calls or text messages.

Experiment with this. Make your list first thing in the morning for several days. Schedule the time. Set an alarm or notification on your phone. Explain to your family what you're doing and how you'll need this time to focus. Then for a couple of days, try making your list at night's end before you go to sleep.

Which method, which scheduled time, seems to be most productive for you? Do you have greater clarity before you go to bed, or do you find yourself more focused first thing in the morning? Each one of us is different, so I want you to decide this for yourself. But you must experiment with this to determine which is best for you, both from the point of clarity and schedule.

Personally, I prefer to create my list in the morning after my workout. I teach a group fitness class most mornings at 5:30. If I don't have a class, I'll meet a friend at the gym or for a run on the trails. On my drive home after a tough workout at the gym, I'm filled with energy. I'm in a great mood and I have a clear mind. When I pull into the driveway, I stay in the car (giving me total solitude) and empty my brain onto my to-do list. I sit quietly. No radio, no sound, still without distractions, I create my task list for the day on my phone. I do this *before* I reenter the house to help get the kids ready and off to school.

(Focus!)

I choose to make my list after my workout because I have found that's when I have the greatest clarity and the least chance of interruption.

If you find it hard to fall asleep at night, I highly suggest making your list at night. You may find you fall asleep faster and wake up with greater clarity.

Step Two: Same Place: Create and Maintain Your To-Do List in Just One Location

The average person creates a to-do list in a multitude of places. Before they leave the office, they slap a stickie note on their computer screen reminding them of the next day's client lunch or afternoon meeting. They write themselves e-mails or create to-do lists on their desktops. The blueprint to their million-dollar-idea is scribbled on a cocktail napkin they carry in their wallet. The mental plan they've created to tackle their fitness goals floats freely in their frontal lobes.

Uh . . . no. That's not cutting it.

Average people create average to-do lists in a variety of places. You're not average. Having only one place you keep and maintain your list is even more important than when you make your list. It's critical to understand how powerful this is.

Think for a moment about where your credit cards and driver's license are. I bet you just slapped your wallet or glanced at your purse.

Daily PUSH

The Roots of My Smartphone Mania

When Bret and I married in 1995, our friend Brian Posey gave us Franklin Covey Day Planners as a wedding gift. Funny how the one thing we didn't have on our wedding registry ended up being the gift that had the greatest impact on our lives together!

I began to write my goals and keep a daily to-do list that year. It wasn't until 2 years later, during my "quest for focus"—and after stumbling upon an ad for a motivational seminar with business and productivity expert Brian Tracy—that I learned to create a frog-eating daily to-do list.

A little more than 12 months after I took his seminar and put his tips into practice, I had achieved nearly every personal *and* professional goal I had set for myself. I began sharing this formula with my personal training clients. The results were encouraging. However, those clients who didn't use a day planner for work, like the stay-at-home moms, found the idea of hauling a planner around inconvenient.

Then digital PDAs hit the market—and, shortly thereafter, the PalmPilot, an early smartphone. These devices allowed users to manage their diets, to-do lists, exercise, calorie journaling, and workout schedules—and this was before apps! I pushed them on my clients with more enthusiasm than I recommended a new set of weights!

Clients and employees who gave in and bought them were soon using them to manage their transformations. Then, in the summer of 2007, Apple introduced the iPhone, and life would never be the same. Enter era of the handheld computer disguised as a smartphone. (Can you hear the angels singing?)

Is there a better place for your to-do list than the device you carry with you every day, all day? You already take your phone just about everywhere you go—to the office, out to dinner, running errands. It's a no-brainer.

You know exactly where to find them because you keep them in the same place, just like your valuable jewels or a family heirloom. You would never mindlessly stash money or jewels around your house, office, or car. We keep track of these things because we recognize their value and importance.

Your daily to-do list is about to become more valuable than all those things put together. Your to-do list is more important than your credit cards, your cash, and your checkbook. I want you to begin treating your to-do list as if it's your retirement fund.

Your daily to-do list will bring you far greater wealth and more free time than anything else you will touch today. You must know where it is and have it with you at all times.

From this day forward, you'll only have one to-do list, and you'll know exactly where it is.

Step Three: Keep Your List with You at All Times

Software developers have created programs to help you be more productive and focused when you're sitting in front of your computer. Great, except that's not all of us. That's not even *most* of us. You have a life outside of your desktop, and I hope you're working to spend less time in front of that computer screen and more time enjoying all that life has to offer. If you're thinking of your to-do list only in terms of remembering tasks and increasing productivity, well, you've missed the point.

This to-do list will *change your life*. It's about creating happiness and reducing stress. It defines your future! That's why you'll want it with you at all times—and it will be, if it's on your smartphone. At some point, it becomes more than a to-do list—it becomes your coach, your accountability, and your map. When you check your e-mail or calendar, you'll check your list, too. And when that fabulous idea strikes, you won't worry about forgetting it. You'll add it to the list and put your mind at ease.

Plus, because your list is with you, you'll have the instant gratification of checking off an item as done. Studies show that we experience an adrenaline rush and a surge of confidence when we feel a sense of accomplishment. Imagine feeling that rush multiple times a day!

Of course, step three is possible only if you're following through on step two: having your to-do list in one location, i.e., your smartphone. Even if you're bullishly stubborn against this whole smartphone thing (for now), at least promise me you will create your list in a place that is small enough and convenient enough for you to have it with you at all times.

But I'm gonna be bossy about treating yourself to a smartphone. You need it. How quickly could you get through the important things in your day and have more time to relax? This is why I'm encouraging you to be open minded enough to make this happen. Get a phone. Put your list on your phone. Make your list the first thing that you see each time you power up. I guarantee this will give you a focus you never imagined.

Step Four: Complete Three Tasks Per Day That Relate to Your "Goals"

When you take small steps toward your goals every day, you're implementing a plan of action and activating momentum toward success. For our purposes, you'll add two or three items each day that move you toward your Push goal and three steps toward your health goal.

In creating your master brainstorm, you've already broken down your big goal into bite-size pieces. You're already in the fast lane.

Never underestimate the impact of small steps. By taking just three small steps every single day toward your goals, you'll create a momentum so powerful that others will stand up and take notice.

Step Five: Revisit and Review Several Times Per Day

Regardless of how focused and well-tuned your memory, distractions arise. You'll need to check your list throughout the day and review what you've accomplished. Give yourself some positive feedback (the adrenaline rush of a checkmark) and blast through the few remaining items. By getting to the most impact-creating actions first, you'll be able to "shut down" sooner. Long gone will be the days of running ragged all day only to ask yourself, "What have I done?"

Referring to your to-do list makes time management effortless. When you check back on your list, you're able to stay focused on the things that must get done, and that's what separates successful people from those who are simply dreamers distracted by being busy. It's very easy to sit down at the computer, find yourself on a Web site that has nothing to do with your goals or your dreams, and waste hours of your time in which you could have easily completed one, two, three, four, or even five tasks on your list. That's the secret of those people who make you wonder how they get it all done.

When someone knows what needs to be done but falls short, it is said they either fear success or they lack the habit of discipline. To be focused, you must keep your eye on the prize. I don't believe that anyone fears success. I believe they have never learned the discipline it takes to achieve it. Focus requires a system that helps us quiet distractions and keep us on task.

The easiest way to stay on task is the habit of checking your list once every hour. Learn to feel the rush of instant gratification each time you check something off your list. We've all done it—added something to our list that we've already done just so we could have the satisfaction of checking it off. It's amazing: You'll experience a rush of endorphins and a confidence-boosting sense of accomplishment that will motivate you to stay on track.

When you get in the habit of checking your list several times a day, a habit triggered simply by the sight of your smartphone, you realize what control you have of your destiny, how much easier it is to manage your time, how much easier it is to get important things done, and, ultimately, how to stay focused. When we're able to stay focused and accomplish the things that we set out to do each day, we feel a sense of self-control. Psychologists generally agree that a sense of control is the key to feeling worthy, to feeling happy, to feeling confident. Those feelings will comfort and reward you in a way far more profoundly than food ever could.

The Power of the Frog (True Story!)

More than a year after committing to align priorities with my goals and then to align my daily to-do list with my Push goal, I remembered that I had listed and sealed a piece of paper with my top-10 objectives in a white business envelope. It was June 2001 when I finally stumbled upon that

Daily PUSH

1. Decide on a time of day to make your list and try it for 1 week before trying an alternative time.

2. Set an alarm on your phone to remind yourself to make your list.

3. Set an alarm on your phone to check your list at least _____ times per day.

NOTES

_____

_____

_____

_____

_____

_____

envelope. There it was, tucked under a pile of T-shirts, in a drawer I rarely opened. I literally gasped. I had forgotten all about it! I was so excited to see it! I ripped it open, eager to see which of my "goals" had been achieved. One by one, number by number, as I read each line the hair on my arms rose up with goose bumps as I realized that so much had been achieved.

My business profits had far exceeded what, at the time, seemed outlandish. We had been able to buy a newer used car without financing. Bret had quit his job, and we were now working together from home. Our marriage and relationship had strengthened in ways I never imagined. Immediately after I created that list, I learned I was pregnant. We had the baby, a girl, and we named her Cierra. Expanding our family had been my first priority. I started to cry when I read what I had written in parentheses: Have a healthy baby girl! Now my eyes were filled with tears, making it difficult to read the list.

Every single goal, one through nine, had been achieved, and more, in less than a year's time. There was only one item not yet accomplished, and ironically it was my number 10: "Buy a big house with a humongous yard!" You see, the reason I had stumbled upon that envelope in the bottom of a rarely opened drawer was because on this day I was packing its contents to move. Yes, we were moving to a much bigger house with that humongous yard. It had taken slightly more than a year to achieve that last item on the list, but we had done it.

Since that time, I have followed a blueprint for the American dream. Nothing gives me more pride than to call myself a happily married mother of two, but it's pretty cool to be introduced as a self-made millionaire. In the words of comedian Chris Rock, "Being rich isn't about the big car or the nice house, it's about options."

Once I refined my own system of to-do list maintenance and took advantage of the technology available to develop this system, most of my 12-month goals are now achieved in 6 months. I have far greater focus, free time, and control over my life. My to-do list has given me lots of options.

By organizing and keeping your to-do list with the focus on your priorities and goals, you will refine your time management and learn to attend to what really matters first. That feeling of being busy all day without accomplishing much will be a distant memory. You too will become a believer, an evangelist for to-do lists. I'm looking forward to your tweets!

Do I have you excited about this? I hope so. And like most really smart people, you probably have a few more specific questions that I can answer for your and make this even more doable! Read on!

TO-DO LIST
Secret Sauce
(Sssshh!)

The Difference Is in the Details

Today I'll give you the recipe for my to-do list secret sauce. The secret sauce adds the "whoa!" factor (yes, "whoa!" not "wow") and takes your list making from something you do to keep yourself organized and transforms it into a handheld GPS: destination success!

If you're totally down with this, if you've said, "Hey, what do I have to lose?" you're my kinda peep. I love ya already. Those who are not willing to try something different will stand staring blankly in a cloud of your dust, baby! God, this is freaking *great!* So assuming you're like me, you need precise details. You want to know exactly what to put on your list, how to organize and prioritize it, and all of the what-ifs that really smart people ask. You'll know by the end of this chapter.

What Goes on Your List

Simple. If needs to be done, it goes on your list. If you need to remember, it goes on your list. If it's a fleeting thought that you need to explore later, a call you need to return, or an e-mail you've just read that you don't have time to respond to at this moment, it goes on your list. You're taking it out of your brain and into the realm of action.

Create One All-Encompassing List

You have one life, right? So you need one to-do list. Yours will include both personal and professional tasks, goals, hopes, dreams, as well as everything in between.

Using one list creates simplicity. I experimented with one list for work, a separate list for errands and projects, and yet another list for fitness pursuits, and quite frankly, it just overcomplicated things. Keep it simple.

Start with an Unloading Dock

When you make your list each day, start at the unloading dock. To "unload" is to spend a few minutes brainstorming every possible task you can think of for today, this month, this year . . . whatever is weighing on your brain.

You see, unconsciously carrying the burden of future tasks creates a level of stress in most of us that can poison our relationships, make us irritable, and cause us to lose sleep. So unload it! Taking these things from your brain to a safe place will help you reduce stress better than a 90-minute massage!

Some days, you'll come up with just a few new tasks. Other days, you'll have so much going on that you spend 15 minutes unloading. Though I want you to create only one list, I do ask you to create four subcategories to help you prioritize activities. Just because you've thought of it today doesn't mean that it should take priority today. Subcategories will help you quickly prioritize your most effective use of time. I use four subcategories: *Today, This Week, This Month, This Year.* I will explain them in detail in just a moment.

At 7:00 a.m., when I create the foundation for my list, I unload everything onto my phone in a category that I label "Today." This is my safety net. After I've unloaded, I can later move items to a less urgent subcategory.

Create Brainstorms and Long Lists on Paper

It makes sense that some of us feel more clarity when we think on paper, especially when we're creating lengthy lists or when we're really on a roll and we find we can write faster than we can type. I actually recommend you create your brainstorm on paper or even use your desktop computer as your unloading dock. But don't forget to e-mail that list, open it on your phone, and copy and paste it into an app or memo. I'm all for creating your master brainstorms and even doing some serious typing on a keyboard bigger than a matchbook, but ultimately the list must be transferred to your phone.

On certain days when there's so much going on and I just can't get my ideas down fast enough, I do exactly that: I take out a very sharp pencil and a legal pad and I go to town creating. But I always transfer it to my phone.

Categorize Your List

There are many elaborate systems for prioritizing to-do lists. I think it's one of the reasons why so many people have negative connotations associated with creating lists. I use a much more manageable hierarchy to roughly prioritize my tasks. Remember, if it wasn't supersimple and snappy fast, I wouldn't do it!

TODAY This category includes things that must be done today or there will be serious consequences. I try not to overwhelm myself with tasks that would be "nice" to accomplish. "Today" specifies the items that absolutely have to be done before I go to bed. Always include three small, very-quick-to-complete tasks that move you toward your Push goal and three tasks that relate to your health goal. In addition to that, list anything that *must* be done. Avoid the temptation to list any item that you'd love to get to if you have time. That's a surefire way to set yourself up for disaster. Those items have a place, and that is in the next category.

THIS WEEK In this section, place the tasks that need to be accomplished by the end of the week. You'll place tasks on your This Week list that you might even like to get to today if you have extra time, but only after you've accomplished three things toward your Push and health goals. I place items in this category that I hope to get done in the next couple of days.

THIS MONTH This is where I put the tasks that I want to accomplish sometime in the near future, perhaps even just a few weeks from now.

THIS YEAR I use this category for things I hope to address in the next 12 months. Remember that these are tasks, projects, and ideas, not goals. Goals need to go on your goals sheet. This category is for items you hope to complete before the year's end. I regularly get overexcited about new ideas when I'm in the unloading mode. It's not uncommon for me to realize some of the projects I've added have no room in my current schedule and belong on my This Year list until I have more room for them. You'll also use this category to house many of the small steps you created in your master brainstorm.

Categories simply allow you to make places to house important ideas. It's not a science. Don't get freaky about this. Just get it out of your head and onto your list!

Going App-Happy

Whether you have a BlackBerry, Droid, Evo, iPhone, Samsung, or some other smartphone, most all smartphones are equipped with their own to-do list software. In the spirit of full disclosure, I am relatively new iPhone convert. I joined the cult a little more than a year before writing this book, and, at print time, I'm happy to report I'm still madly in love.

Before my latest iPhone love affair, I was a bit promiscuous with my smartphone relationships. The good news is that I can tell you firsthand this system works on any phone with the ability to text. At the moment I'm loving an iPhone app called Awesome Note, but I often try new ones, so be sure to check my Web site for the latest app recommendations according to brand.

How you use your app is very individual. I'm visual, so I need an app that quickly displays icons and category names. I also need an app that syncs to my desktop computer and allows me or my team to access my list remotely via Evernote. This allows me to see my team's lists, and they see mine. Think of your app in the same way you would think of a day planner. A particular size, function, and certain features may make one brand a better fit for your lifestyle. Apps typically cost $1 or less. What the heck, spend 5 bucks and do some app testing for yourself.

Calendaring Tasks

Many people ask if you should attach due dates to your tasks. My opinion is *only when absolutely necessary.* Adding one more step, even though it may only take 30 seconds, will diminish your discipline to stick to this formula. Remember, this system is about speed and convenience. The only time I add a date is when it's a pending task that I may have placed on my This Week or This Month list and I want to remind myself to start in advance. In that event, I simply add an alert or an alarm to my phone several weeks or days out. One of the best time-saving features of using your phone is that you'll never have to transfer or rewrite tasks to the next day or week.

I suspect that there are some of you who believe that you've done very well for yourself keeping your list on a legal pad or your day planner. Perhaps you believe that using the tiny keypad on your phone is too cumbersome. I hear ya; I'm a big fan of taking pen to paper. Something magical can happen with a sharpened pencil and a crisp new legal pad.

My father-in-law is one of the most organized and fit 65-plus dudes I know. He has never used a smartphone. Coincidentally, he's been following my system of keeping a to-do list almost to a T; the only exception is that he doesn't use his phone. He carries a yellow legal pad everywhere he goes. And you know what, that's okay! He's following the most important steps: keeping it with him at all times, checking it several times a day, creating it in the same location every time, and making his list at the same time each day. There are exceptions. But keep in mind, he spends a great deal of time transferring tasks from one page to a new page. He has no way of backing up his legal pad, and sometimes it's just a bit inconvenient to lug that thing around, but he does it!

Save Time by Not Having to Rewrite Tasks

Your phone allows those things that you did not complete today to transfer to the next day's list. Though transferring your initial brainstorm may take a few extra minutes, the time it will save you in the long run is immeasurable. Sometimes you have to slow down to speed up. This one step will save you ten in the long run.

Slow Down to Speed Up

Warning: I'm going to make my case for a smartphone . . . again! It's not that I think you missed it the first five times I made my case for you to transition your organization to your smartphone. Rather, as an optimist, I'm going to assume you simply need a reminder. I know you're busy with a vast array of responsibilities. I imagine someone as sharp as you has been thinking very seriously about it. Perhaps distractions have prevented you from having the time to look into pricing or revising your cellular plan. It could be that your biggest concern is finding the time to learn a new phone's features. Whatever you *say* is the reason, it's just an excuse. Excuses do two things: 1) They help you stay in your comfort zone. 2) They prevent you from living the life that you really want.

No more making the excuse that you don't have time to figure out a new phone or that you can't afford to upgrade from your current phone. You're waiting until your plan allows you to upgrade for free. You think you should wait until the next update comes out. Money is tight.

Sorry. I love ya, I really do, but you and I both know that the life you want is worth finding a way. Be resourceful! You can sell a few things on eBay and buy a refurbished smartphone for practically pennies to make all of this possible. This is

1. Download one or two to-do list apps.

2. Create four subcategories (exactly or similar to the concept explained above).

3. Now begin placing tasks in the appropriate file or category.

NOTES

_____

_____

_____

_____

_____

_____

_____

an investment. This is not a toy. If you're serious about getting your life in shape, you need to spend your money wisely. So . . . what do you say? Is it time for a new phone?

If your current phone is driving you bonkers, get rid of it. I'm telling you this from personal experience. The last phone I had drove me crazy. I kept it for months and just kept complaining about how difficult it was to keep my to-do list on it. I had switched from a phone that I loved to one that everyone told me to get. It totally didn't work for me. I kept explaining to people, "I can't get a new phone, I just got this one." Dumb answer.

Then it dawned on me. How much is my time worth? How much do I value the functionality of my to-do list? I couldn't put a price on that. The most valuable thing I own is my to-do list. So I smacked myself upside my head and took my own advice. Even though it wasn't time to upgrade, I made that investment in my own peace of mind. In doing so, I saved myself, literally, dozens of hours in frustration and became more focused by using a phone that allowed me the simplicity I like when it comes to my to-do list. Take the time and invest in a smartphone that ultimately could change your life.

Successful people recognize that learning new technology requires an investment of time. So go ahead and set aside the time to learn it, master it, and allow it to work to your advantage. Know that your investment of time will save you tenfold in the long run. Regardless of where you decide to create your to-do list, make sure it's with you at all times.

You've already created some incredible habits: the habit of creating a daily to-do list, the habit of adding two or three items to your list that pertain to your Push goal. Every time you add an item to your list or check your list, you're then thinking about your Push goal. And, as we know, your thoughts become your reality: Whatever you think about most starts to become your reality, and that's why you're gaining so much momentum.

DAY 11
Your **SOUL-MATE** Workout

Be Open to Finding Love!

Today I'm going to play cupid and help you fall head over heels in love with a workout perfectly suited for just you!

Most people, even those who don't enjoy exercise, have at least one workout they consider "tolerable." You might even be one of those lucky human types who almost enjoys exercise.

Whichever the case maybe, I want you to experience something much more profound. I want you to experience love.

My goal today is to help you define what you're looking for in a soul mate. Your assignment will be to tap into what gives you joy and makes you feel alive and then narrow down your search. Together, through a series of simple exercises, you'll understand that we can find an exercise program so well suited for you that you'll feel addicted and beg for more! You'll go from thinking of exercise as tolerable or even

enjoyable to one that will have you flipping over backwards, head over heels in love with "your" workout.

Scoff if you must. The proof is in the numbers. I've been able to help millions of former couch potatoes turn into raving lunatics for exercise. And here's the truth . . . I don't care if it's my workout, or some form of outdoor activity, or some crazy thing you invent on your own. Anyone who says there's only one perfect exercise is only thinking of himself or herself.

When it comes to love, you're unique and must find your own unique life partner. The same is true for your cardio workout.

So relax. Smile. Be open to finding love.

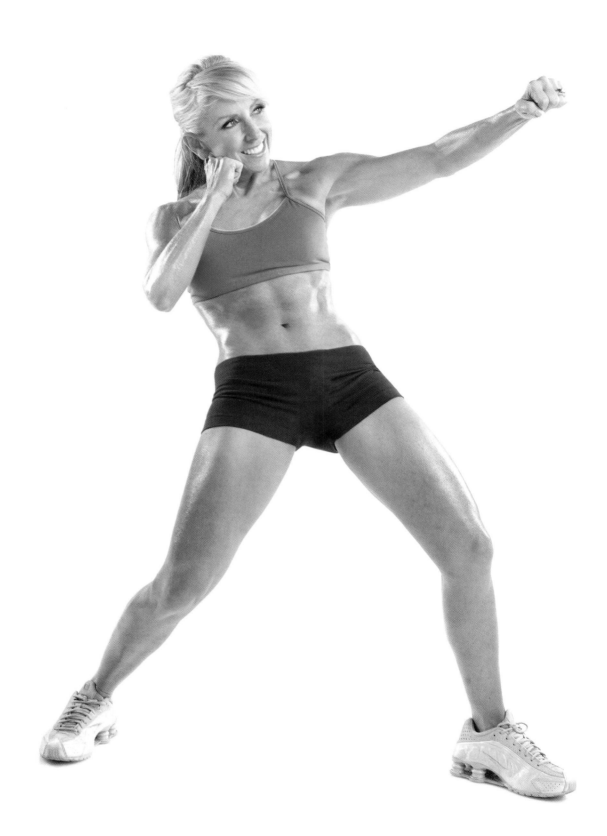

Searching for "the One"

It is said that when you meet the love of your life, you'll feel a spark and know immediately you were meant to be together. Your soul mate is that person to whom you are drawn in a way you've never experienced before; a love so deep you can't get enough. When you've met your soul mate, you wonder how you ever thought you were once in love with someone other than this cosmically perfect person.

Love gives you energy. Love creates a powerful rush of endorphins. The world feels new and excit-ing. New love inspires you to care about yourself, your goals, the impression you're making on oth-ers, your dress, your posture, and even your appearance. Your appetite is distracted by thoughts of planning when you'll next be together. You feel understood. *"Where have you been all my life?"*

If you don't love exercise, it just means you haven't yet met your soul-mate workout. Finding your soul mate is invaluable to your lifelong fit-ness success. When you find your soul-mate workout, you'll have the key ingredient to creat-ing a bangin' body and the life you deserve.

Never give up on love!

If you had a lovely friend who deserved all

(continued on page 80)

How You'll Know You've Found True Love

I want you to know what it feels like when you find your soul-mate workout. With this description as your guide, you'll know if you've found "it" or if you need to keep "dating" workouts!

- ▶ Your soul-mate workout makes you feel you can do anything.
- ▶ Your soul-mate workout challenges you never to be complacent.
- ▶ Your soul-mate workout makes you feel alive, sexy, and young.
- ▶ Your soul-mate workout feels like a treat, even when it's brutal.
- ▶ When you're doing your soul-mate workout, you are surprised by how fast time passes.
- ▶ Your soul-mate workout clears your mind and calms your emotions.
- ▶ You can't help but endlessly talk about your soul-mate workout.
- ▶ Your soul-mate workout awakens your spirit.
- ▶ Your soul-mate workout gives you energy, creativity, and drive.
- ▶ You look forward to your next workout.

Your soul-mate workout is out there, waiting for you to find it.

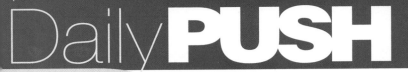

Today's Homework

YOUR SOUL-MATE WORKSHEET

Finding my life soul mate (Bret) was the best thing that ever happened to me personally. Creating my soul-mate workout was the best thing that ever happened to me physically.

Everyone has the potential to fall in love with exercise. That's what your soul-mate workout represents—your love for exercise. Your soul-mate workout is simply a gateway drug! I don't expect you to be monogamous with your soul-mate workout. I want you to know that love can happen and allow yourself to throw open the doors of possibility.

Finding your soul-mate workout can be done in the very same way you might find your soul-mate partner. Begin by thinking about the qualities you're most interested in finding. What do you want in a workout? Once in a while you stumble upon true love, but most often you have to know what you want and go out and find it. The same is true of a workout. Let's get started!

1. Circle your preference of the characteristics below. Then transfer your circled word to the line to the right.

▶ Indoor or outdoor? _____

▶ Group or solo? _____

▶ Team or individual? _____

▶ Dance or athletic? _____

▶ Competitive or noncompetitive? _____

▶ Slow and steady or fast and furious? _____

▶ High-impact, low-impact, or nonimpact? _____

▶ Music or silence? _____

▶ Very coordinated, somewhat coordinated, or two left feet? _____

_____

2. Answer the questions below.

▶ The sport you enjoy the most is:_____

▶ What were you doing the last time you felt young and alive while exercising? _____

_____

▶ What types of exercise do you find mundane or torturous? _____

_____

▶ What kind of music inspires you? _____

▶ In what kind of environment do you find you work the hardest? Group? Solo? On a team?

_____

_____

▶ What types of activities or sports did you most enjoy in your youth? _____

_____

▶ Do you work out harder or with greater intensity when in the presence of others? _____

_____

▶ Is fashion and people watching interesting to you? _____

▶ Do you need an opportunity to clear your mind and be alone? _____

▶ Do you meditate? _____

▶ If you could go back in time and have really mastered a sport or activity, what would that be?

_____

▶ What sport or activity do you enjoy watching on TV?_____

_____

3. Reread the list of adjectives you've transferred to the right-hand column. Now reread your replies to the list of questions above and, together, summarize the type of exercise or activities you might have described. In some instances, you might be inventing your own:

_____

_____

_____

_____

_____

_____

_____

4. You're going to date your workout now. Don't worry, this is gonna be fun. Even the worst dates teach you something about yourself. Dating workouts will add zest to your weekly routine and maybe even give you a chuckle. As I always say, "Mistakes burn calories, too!"

List the types of activities you hereby commit to "trying" in the next 7 days.

_____

_____

_____

_____

_____

_____

_____

This is not junior high PE. If you're not good at something on your first day, no one is going to judge you. No one is good at something on the first try. Lose the ego and learn to enjoy.

When trying something new, everyone feels a little bit like an idiot. No one ever died from embarrassment. But it doesn't hurt to do a little prep work before your first date.

Don't be afraid to ask for help. Make things easier on yourself by calling ahead and finding out what you need to succeed.

- ▶ What to wear
- ▶ What to expect
- ▶ How to best prepare
- ▶ How much it costs
- ▶ What kind of equipment you need

A little advance information will make the experience much more pleasant. If you go for a spinning class without bringing a padded seat, you're going to regret it the next day when you try to sit down. Ask to borrow one from a friend. Actually, asking a friend to share his or her passion about a workout is a great way to try something new. Be open and willing to learn.

As you're learning to think of yourself as an athlete, trying new things won't be outside of your normal experience. When you get a chance to learn a new sport, take it! Ask friends what workouts they enjoy and invite yourself along.

For the next few months, it would be a reasonable goal to try something new every week. Once you've found your soul-mate workout, you're going to want to connect with it. But even then, continue to explore. Athletes love a challenge!

that life had to offer, yet she always picked the wrong guy to fall in love with, you wouldn't tell her to give up on love! Most of us date a few frogs before we find our prince.

Recently, I asked my friends on Facebook to describe what it was like to finally meet their soul mates. Here's what they said:

Rachel Gonzales Knew almost immediately. I loved it because of the "party" atmosphere. Feel like a rockstar after every workout; feel incomplete when have to skip it and then can't wait to make it up. Always look forward to do it again; wanna share with everyone. Guess it's just like when u have that first puppy love.

Be a Fool for Love!

Trying something new, no matter how nervous, awkward, and foolish you feel at first, will give you confidence in the long run.

A couple years ago, I was in Park City, Utah, snowboarding with my family. From the window of our hotel, I could see a field of cross-country skiers. I remarked to Bret that it must be a killer workout because absolutely every skier was fit and lean! I had to try it!

So the next morning I went down and rented myself a pair of cross-country skis and some poles. This being my first attempt, all that I had to wear was my oversize, outrageously bright pair of snowboarding pants along with my equally wild jacket and floppy hat. Add to that my rhinestone-blinged goggles and you've got yourself a real fish out of water. I might as well have worn a big sign around my neck that said "I have no idea what I'm doing!"

I must have looked like a total buffoon to the cross-country skiers in their skintight black tights and muted sweaters. I really stood out. I stepped my skis into a set of tracks and started on my way. I didn't get very far before I fell over like an overstuffed Michelin man. My skis were still in the tracks. I was up and down, up and down all morning, but my iPod was pumping great tunes and I was sweating like never before.

Sure, it was a little embarrassing to jump out of the way so that a 10-year-old skier could navigate his way around me, but it was a killer workout!

I signed up for a lesson the next morning. I explained that I was a beginner (as if I needed to state the obvious!). And sure enough, with a little guidance and a little patience with myself, I learned the basics of cross-country skiing.

Keri Gross Running . . . I had never been a runner and envied anyone who was but when I was overweight, I never thought it was something I would ever be able to accomplish. After losing over 75 pounds, I decided to "try" it and now I am an avid runner after only a year into it. I'm addicted and I love the way it makes me feel!!! :) Anyone who has the ability to run should! Wonderful stress release and it makes me feel alive and amazing. Ran 7 yesterday. Plan to run 7 tomorrow too :)

 Gabby Whitney My soulmate workout hooked me during the first try. The characteristics that drew me in: 1) different than all the rest, 2) difficult without being unnecessarily impossible, 3) incorporates interval overload followed by quick relief stretching. It feels empowering, graceful, and I've never plateaued. I feel strong and accomplished and energetic and relaxed on days I do these workouts. On days I don't, I actually miss it. It's hard to take a day off!

Daily**PUSH**

In addition to the two tasks that relate to your Push goal, add the two physical tasks below that move you toward your health goal. Don't forget to add two simple tasks that relate to nutrition.

1. Take a look at the list you've completed and the adjectives you carried over to the right side column. Read those comments in succession. What workouts come to mind?

2. Schedule a date and time to try a new workout.

3. Do your research. Find out what you should wear, expect, bring, or how best to prepare for your first date.

NOTES

_____

_____

_____

_____

How I Found *My* Soul-Mate Workout

Maybe you've thought to yourself, "If I could find a guy with Steve's sense of humor, Jon's drive, Randy's sweet side, but Luke's wild streak and could mix that with some of Joe's height and Todd's good looks, I'd have the perfect man!"

In much the same way many reflect on the qualities of lovers past, I want you to look back on the qualities of past exercise and leisure activities. Think about what you're looking for in an exercise. That's what I did to create my perfect workout. I come from an active family. I learned to ski at age 4, ride motocross at 5, and horseback ride at 7. We spent our summers on a lake. We swam, ran the trails, water-skied, and rode bikes. I played golf and ran cross-country. I took jazz, tap, and ballet lessons. I tried gymnastics, basketball, volleyball, track, and softball. I was a cheerleader for a couple of years (shocker, I know). I tried my hand at martial arts. At the gym, I tried yoga, step classes, cycling, and even high-impact aerobics.

They were okay. I enjoyed their company. But truly, I hadn't yet met my soul mate. My sister Jenelle, on the other hand, fell in love with ballet very young. She came alive when she danced. Just a few chords on the piano and she transformed. She wanted to spend every waking moment in ballet. Even as a teen, she'd rush home, change into her pale pink tights and tattered leg warmers, grab her pointe shoes, and whisk off to dance. For hours she'd practice, until her feet were swollen and bleeding. We loved to watch her dance. You could see in her eyes that she was in love.

It's the same spark you'd see in my father's hazel green eyes just before he slapped shut the plastic eye shield on his helmet, smiled, and raced off into the woods on his motorcycle. He'd come back sweaty, dirty, exhausted, and happy beyond measure.

I wanted to feel that.

Desperate for that feeling, I decided to take matters into my own hands and create my own workout. (Insert *Weird Science* music here.) I created my soul mate.

I loved the music of hip hop, the athleticism of volleyball, the results from running, the superhero power of tae kwon do, and the hip shaking of freestyle dance. I mixed that with the sound effects from my cheerleading days and *BAM*—I had *my* soul-mate workout!

Little did I know that my workout fusion would appeal to others who were looking for the same. I created a soul mate for me. And you can create yours!

When people first caught wind of this workout I had created, Turbo Kick, they would say things like, "That's not hip hop," "You're not supposed to shake your hips when you do a boxing speedbag," "That's not a tae kwon do back kick." To which I would reply, "*So? I* like it. If I can get people to move, have fun, sweat buckets, and fall in love with exercise, who gives a rat's ass what the rules are?!?"

So you want to dance while you run? Do it! You want to ride a stationary bike while practicing your tennis serve? Go for it. You'd love golfing if you could run between holes and jog through your swing? What have you got to lose?!?

SUCCESSORIZING

Must-Have Weight-Loss Weapons

Look, it doesn't cost a dime to lose weight. Watch *Survivor* or go a few days without enough money to buy food and you'll know that's a fact! And ya know what? You don't need a computer to run a business. But if you're serious about success, you invest in the right tools!

Times are tough. Money is tight. I'm not suggesting that you *have* to buy a bunch of gadgets, but it's my job to give you the edge and help you make informed decisions about your investments. And the truth is, the right tools—some of which you may already own—save you time, establish accountability, get you motivated, and build your foundation. You wouldn't trust a home constructed by a builder with makeshift tools.

Remember when you were a kid, how excited you were about your new clothes and cool lunchbox for the first day of school? Or how cool it was to move into your first apartment and buy your first broom, ladder, and laundry hamper? First day of school, first year out on your own, empirically both scary. You weren't scared; you were excited about your new "stuff," a fresh start, a

chance to reinvent yourself. The tools make your journey easier, more exciting, and convenient. The right tools make your success more likely.

Weight-loss tools spark enthusiasm, the fuel your spirit needs. I've listed them in order of impact. That is to say, the items at the top of the list have been proven to have the most dramatic impact on the success of the people I work with. Spend your money wisely. Each of these investments you can expect to use daily.

1. Diet and Exercise Journal or App

You already know I'm a big fan of anything that fits conveniently into the palm of your hand.

The more convenient, the more likely we are to adopt the habit of accurate calorie and exercise journaling. Your smartphone is really the way to go! However, some really great sites also provide free journaling tools and community accountability, such as SparkPeople.com, Teambeachbody.com, and Livestrong.com.

In terms of physically taking a pen to paper, I LOVE the Fitbook! It's simple, inclusive, small, and easy to use! (Visit www.getfitbook.com.) I've listed your journal or journaling app as the most important tool. However, it's only effective if it's used as an honest record keeper. Um, and yes, those two last bites of Johnnie's pancakes need to be recorded! When in doubt, round up!

2. Personal Calorie-Monitoring Device

You need to create a deficit of 3,500 calories to lose a pound. The problem is, most people have no idea how many calories they have to burn to create that deficit unless they know how many calories they (with all their individual variables) burn per day.

Research has shown that the average person overestimates the calories he or she burns by 25 percent and underestimates the number consumed by 40 percent! Don't be that person!

You can track your calories for free with varying degrees of accuracy using a number of free sites listed on page 279. However, if money is not an issue and accuracy is, these monitoring devices are *remarkable!* Other than living in a lab, this is about the best way to know what's going on with your personal metabolism, sleep patterns, and caloric burn.

Keep in mind there's a big difference between a digital calorie-monitoring device and a heart rate monitor. I'm talking about a device that measures calorie output. The price keeps going down, and the accuracy continues to improve. Think of them as a metabolism monitor and truth detector all in one!

When people say to me, "Chalene, I'm doing everything right, I've reduced my calories, I'm exercising every day, and I just can't lose weight," I strongly encourage them to get one of these devices. I've seen hundreds of men and women break long-lasting weight-loss plateaus by "knowing their numbers." When I started wearing a calorie monitor just a few years ago, I was shocked by how much I was overestimating my calorie burn in certain exercises and underestimating my daily activity rate. The information allowed me to restructure my workout schedule to get the most bang for my buck. Call me a gadget geek, but these things fascinate me!

- Fitbit—www.fitbit.com. Love the simplicity, small size, accurate info; there's no need for an additional subscription or digital display to read your information.

- GoWear Fit—www.amazon.com. Made by the same company as the Bodybugg (see below), but with slightly different software and customer support system.

- Bodybugg—www.bodybugg.com. This is the calorie-monitoring device worn by contestants of *The Biggest Loser* television show. I've worked with several contestants once they've been sent home to prepare for their final weigh-in on the finale show. I fell in love with the Bodybugg technology and the level of customer support. Less expensive, less technical options are out there, but this one (at time of print) is my current pick!

3. Portable Food Containers

When it comes to preparation, convenience is the key. You need the following sizes and quantities:

- Two ½-cup containers. This size is perfect for most of the Throw-and-Go concoctions in the recipe section.
- Four 1-cup containers. These hold ½ cup of brown rice and 5 ounces of chicken.
- Two ¼-cup containers. These work well for sauces and condiments.

I know you've probably seen this thing or something like it advertised on TV or on the shelf at your local discount store and wondered if they work. *They do!* As a matter of fact, I bought 20 sets last year and gave them away to all my fit-minded friends! You can find them at a variety of online retailers for between $9.95 and $19.95. I love the neat and tidy stackable system of Smart Spin Storage brand, but any brand will do!

4. The George Foreman Grill

Will any fat grilling machine work? Sure. But I've tried most of them. Let me save you some time and money and tell you good ol' Georgie boy makes the best! I've had every variety of countertop grill in the last 10 years and nobody makes one better!

Now, here's why you need one. Even if you often cook on your stovetop or you think you'd beat Bobby Flay in a BBQ Showdown, a countertop grill strips a lot of the fat and cuts the preparation time down to mere minutes. In 5 minutes flat (less time than what you will spend wandering through your cupboards looking for something processed and crunchy because you are hungry RIGHT NOW), you can have a fresh breast of grilled chicken, grilled asparagus, and ½ cup of brown rice.

5. Exercise DVDs

No, this is not a shameless plug for my own DVDs! Rather, this is to suggest that when you have a library of fitness DVDs, you always have options on hand. If you haven't tried an exercise DVD in recent years, or you don't think you can get a good workout at home, guess again.

Seven years ago, I partnered with fitness infomercial folks Beachbody to bring my health club workout to consumers. What I love about Beachbody's approach to fitness is that it's real. They don't sugarcoat anything. If you want a kick-ass body, you need a kick-ass workout. They are by far the best in the industry, bar none, and I'm not just speaking about my own products offered by Beachbody, but all of their workouts! There's something for everyone, and the programs are researched, tested, and produced to the highest standards.

Exercise DVDs are perfect for exercising on

the road, during inclement weather, or when you're just in the mood to have someone else motivate you! Whether it's an athletic workout, cycling, dance, plyometrics, speed and agility, or ethnic dance, there's a DVD to foot the bill.

6. Measuring Devices

Good news! You probably already have most of these—measuring cups, a digital food scale, and measuring spoons. Now it's a matter of putting them in a place where you will see them (and use them) every day. Remember, this is about creating convenient, second-nature habits. I keep my own measuring devices in a drawer under the exact spot on the counter I use for my own food prep each day.

Weigh and measure all food for 30 days. At the end of 30 days, you'll be a pro at sizing up portions and you'll be able to relax this practice. However, once a year, I ask you to spend 1 week back in this practice. Portions left unchecked over time get larger and larger. Every once in a while, do a little personal quality control inspection!

7. Portable Music Device and Playlist

Music is a universal motivator. Music boosts your spirits and gives you energy. Music motivates us to do more and push harder. If you have a smartphone that allows you to download killer selections, instead of buying a portable music device such as an iPod, invest $10 and 20 min-

utes creating an electrifying playlist for your phone. Daily, someone sends me a message asking how to find the motivation to exercise, and this is undoubtedly my go-to answer.

8. Exercise Tubing

Tubing is the bomb! You must have a set of tubing or exercise bands (often the two terms are used interchangeably) for travel purposes. I also love the affordability of tubing for those who are looking to build a home gym on a budget. They can be just as effective as using free weights while requiring virtually zero space. Choke up on the band to create a heavier resistance, or adjust to make them feel lighter! They're economical, lightweight, and easy to use.

Exercise bands can create the same resistance created by free weights. They look harmless, but they work! Your bicep doesn't care whether the force created is from a band or a weight. Though admittedly I love the feel of working with free weights, they are very expensive and require some space.

Don't buy crappy bands at a discount store, though! They don't last. I love the durability of the tubing offered through Beachbody.com as well as SPRI, Inc. Beachbody includes its tubing in many of its deluxe workout DVD systems, and SPRI offers a Traveling Trainer kit. This easy, safe, and effective program kit comes complete with three SPRI Deluxe Xertube products of varied resistance, a door attachment, a 26-minute exercise video, an exercise instructional guide, a diner's guide, and Michael Sena's personal training workout programs. The kit runs approximately $50.

9. Emergency Food

I think it would be superfreaking fantastic if you farmed your own sugarcane, breakfast was fresh berries from your organic garden, and your children drank water from the stream on the mountaintop where you lived in your log cabin constructed entirely of recycled paper products. But let's get real.

By this point, you understand that I believe the "lesser of two evils" approach to food is more realistic than professed perfection. *Of course* unprocessed is the way to go. Duh! But unless you have a full-time assistant following you around, you need an emergency plan. Despite your best planning, there will be plenty of moments when you have 5 minutes to get out the door, you haven't eaten, and there's not a piece of fresh food in the house! While unprocessed organic whole food is our goal, that might not be in the cards when you find yourself stuck at the office at 7:00 p.m.

Here are a few things I recommend you always have on hand:

- Top-of-the-line meal replacement shake with protein
- Raw almonds and freeze-dried fruit
- A box of the best engineered protein bars

I shy away from endorsing specific brands of food, though I do have my faves! The choices you make boil down to cost, ingredients, and personal preferences with regard to taste and texture.

I'm sure the food police will send me enough hate mail to fill a room for this suggestion, and I'm not fazed. That's because I've met thousands and thousands of people who, when 100 percent unprocessed perfection wasn't available, believed they had failed their diet and turned to a far worse alternative than a protein shake or protein bar (both of which are processed . . . **oh no** . . . *gasp!*).

It's okay! Permission granted to not be perfect! You need *healthier* options for the days when the *healthiest* of options are unavailable.

When selecting meal replacements (bars or protein powders) choose whey over soy (unless you're vegan or lactose intolerant). Look for brands without additives, as many of the lesser-priced bars and powders are not much more than sawdust! And your healthiest options are 100 percent protein concentrate, not isolate. Just like fresh fruit is more nutritious than canned, there is less processing involved in a concentrate than in an isolate. Vegans might also consider hemp proteins. Though such foods can be difficult to find, every one of us needs an emergency food plan!

10. New Kicks!

What was it about the first day of school that was always so exciting and wonderful? It wasn't all the learning you'd be doing, it was probably because you had a new outfit and really fast new shoes. Not much has changed. In addition to providing you with the proper support and cushion you need for your soul-mate workout, new shoes may also inspire you to put your plan into action.

Studies show that when we feel good about what we're wearing on the job, we work harder and longer. The same is true of our workouts. As for the type of shoe, I don't recommend a particular brand. Every foot is different. Visit a sports retailer with a knowledgeable sales staff who can address your footwear needs.

11. Calorie Reference Guides

Forget trying to memorize or estimate calorie counts; invest in a small portable reference guide that fits neatly into your purse, office drawer, or car console.

For smartphone users, an app is your best bet. You will find the calorie, fat, protein, and carbohydrate counts for your favorite foods according to brand, size, and portion, plus restaurant entrees, fast food, and more! Whether it's the extremely thorough, convenient pocket-size CalorieKing (from CalorieKing.com; $8.50) or a free app like the überpopular Livestrong.com app for iPhone and Android, the difference is in the numbers. Underestimating consumption by as little as 1 ounce per day can result in more than a 10-pound weight gain over the course of a year.

Daily PUSH

While you need none of the aforementioned goodies to "make it happen," if you've got the coin, or you consider your health important enough to forgo a few nonessentials this month, you can't go wrong with treating yourself to any one of them.

1. Shop!

2. Shop!

3. Shop!

NOTES

_____

_____

_____

_____

_____

_____

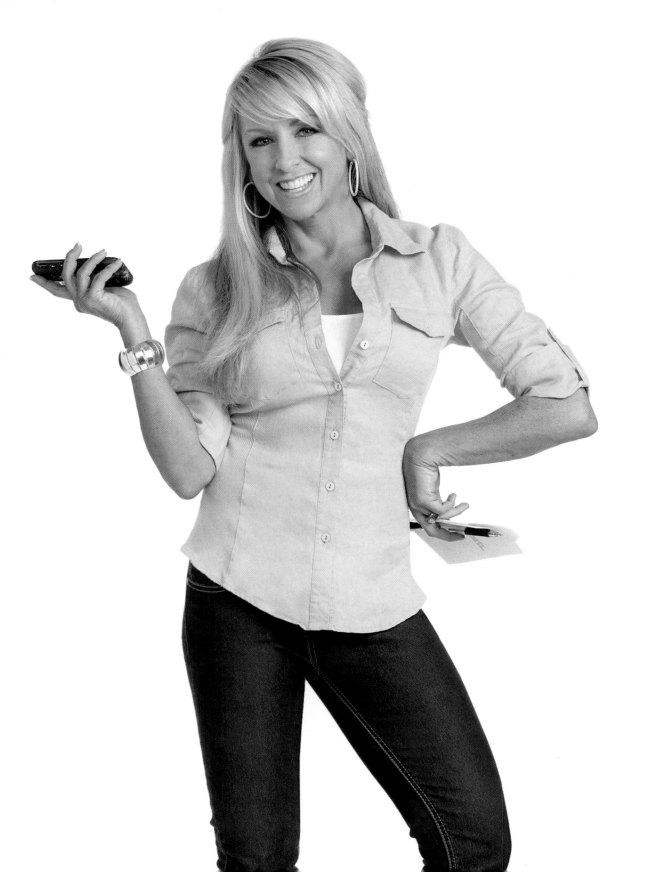

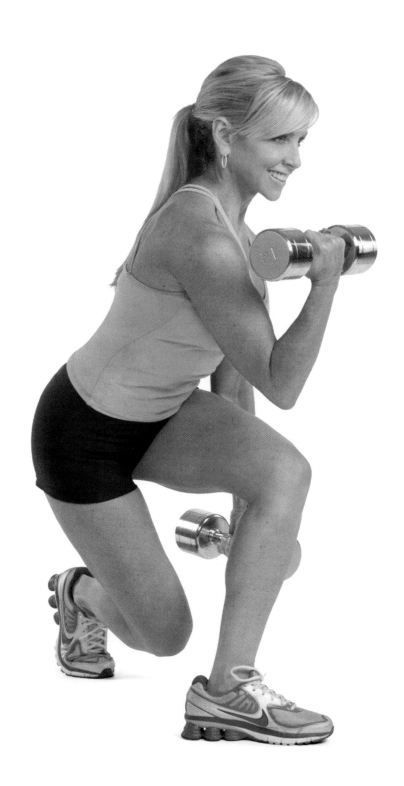

DAY 13

The Bangin'
BODY FORMULA

Everything You Need to Know to Get the Bangin' Body You Deserve

Before we get too far, I want to get ya started building your bangin' body! Today I'm going to share with you "best practices" and a summary of research on the type of program that will provide you with the very best results.

I *am not* giving you a personalized fitness program. I *am* giving you the knowledge you need to customize your own and putting you in charge of your success.

The "Best Workout" Is the One You'll Do

Ultimately, the exercise program that will give you the best results is the one that you'll do with consistency and intensity. For some, the best exercise program might be running and yoga, while a combination of swimming and strength training will work best for others. There's little benefit to prescribing a one-size-fits-all exercise program, because you get the best results when you customize your own.

Oh sure, there's no shortage of well-intentioned personal trainers working their 9:00 a.m. client, a 49-year-old female with chronic knee pain, the same way they train their 5:00 p.m. client, a 27-year-old male with type 2 diabetes. But any trainer worth an hourly rate understands the mountain of variables that should be considered and how they relate uniquely to you.

I could tell you what *I* think will work for *most* people, but I genuinely believe you will be best served by learning the most effective exercise parameters and then blending your own program.

Basic Fitness Facts

In the study of exercise science, there are several universally held principles scientifically proven to provide optimal physical and mental health. *Phew*, that made me sound supersmart—I get like that when I talk fitness. Let me back up and present this in understandable terms. I like science. Science trumps trend any day of the week.

When I set out to create an at-home exercise program or one of the many workouts I've designed for the country's leading health clubs, I always start with science as my foundation. Adding trendy, exciting components to an exercise program is simple, provided you let science be your guide. These components can be reduced to three basic fitness facts that your customized program must include. So consider them as you create your own plan.

1. INDIVIDUAL DIFFERENCES

Everyone is different. One size does not fit all. Individual variables that affect exercise include age, weight, dieting history, genetics, medical conditions, injuries, and, of course, gender, to name a few. For example, women generally need more recovery time than men. A cardio junkie who has hit a plateau needs strength training to build muscle. Long-distance runners might benefit from endurance training as opposed to strength. The best program for one individual might not be as effective for another.

With this in mind, when I create at-home exercise programs, I spend a boatload of time developing options that include instructions for beginners, differing directives for athletes, and special considerations for those with knee and back issues. Regardless of how much concern I devote to individual variables, there is still a pretty good chance that the workouts might not be the right fit for every person who tries them. Even the most comprehensive off-the-shelf exercise program, group fitness class, or DVD set (and I am proud to say programs such as Turbo Fire, Turbo Jam, and ChaLEAN Extreme have set the bar) is best customized by you!

Your customized exercise plan must take into consideration your personal fitness objectives and your unique variables.

2. THE OVERLOAD PRINCIPLE

The overload principle is a process of training that addresses how your body responds to change and incorporates exercises you must do to create improvement. And we're all looking to change for the better, right? To change, your body needs a reason. When the systems of your body take on more "load" (greater intensity, longer duration, or anything that's tougher, more stressful, or even just different from what you've done in the past), the body says, "In the event you do this again, we'll get you ready!"

In other words, to improve your fitness, strength, or endurance, you need to challenge your body accordingly.

In order for a muscle (including the heart) to strengthen, it must be gradually pushed to work harder. By working against a load greater than it is used to via greater intensity, longer duration, or both, the muscles are challenged. Our muscles, yes, even our hearts, rise to the occasion and naturally increase strength.

If change is what you desire, your regular exercise routine must be something that is tougher, longer, or more challenging than what you are doing right now.

3. ADAPTATION AVOIDANCE

Adaptation refers to the body's ability to predict what's coming next. Your magnificent machine adjusts intuitively to meet increased or decreased physical demands. It is one way we learn to coordinate muscle movement and develop sport-specific or dance-specific skills, such as batting, swimming freestyle, mamboing, or shooting free throws. Doing the same exercise, or practicing the same skill or physical activity, makes it easier to perform.

Here's an example of how adaptation influenced my exercise programs. If we want to make certain claims on TV, the FTC requires that we be able to back up our statements with sufficient evidence. My partners at Beachbody pride themselves on producing fitness programs that work and making claims they can substantiate! (Unfortunately, many of the other late-night infomercial companies don't hold themselves to the same standard. Not trying to dog others, it's just fact.) For my *Turbo Jam* infomercial, we conducted doctor-supervised clinical testing to measure caloric expenditure. The test group

included a cross section of the general population (i.e., all sizes, ages, and levels of fitness). Now listen, I knew that if the calorie burn was anywhere close to what I had estimated it to be, this workout program would be a number-one seller! So, as you might expect, I too asked if I could be in the test group. The doctor obliged but suggested that my own results might actually hurt the study. "What?" I thought. "Oh, this guy has no idea how hard I go!"

True confession: I planned to "crush it" on the calorie-testing day. My intention was to kick my own bootay beyond the point of return—to go harder than I have ever done before. I wanted huge, impressive numbers to prove to people how many calories they could burn with this workout! I prepared mentally and nutritionally, got a great night's sleep, and gave my very best effort! My plan didn't go so well.

Here's the irony. Because Turbo was/is my soul-mate workout, the cardio that I had been doing for at least 12 years, my body had fully adapted. Just as the doc predicted, my own caloric burn was in the bottom 25 percent of the test group. Talk about a bummer. Can you say "rude awakening"?

Did this mean that I would have to find a new workout? Nope. But it did mean I needed to change some things, and you might need to as well.

The calorie-testing experience was the catalyst for my need to research and understand exercise adaptation more fully. I set out to tweak my soul-mate workout to overcome adaptation.

To avoid experiencing adaptation, you can add elements, expand duration, increase intensity, and generally create a change of intensity or duration (aka *periodization*) every 30 days. To avoid divorcing my soul mate, I began cycling additional challenges, such as weighted hand gloves and high-intensity interval training. It worked! By having this knowledge and then customizing according to my individual experience, I was able to dramatically improve my own caloric burn and avoid the dreaded exercise plateau that results when your body adapts to your regular routine.

Change elements of intensity, duration, or overall challenge in your regular program to avoid exercise adaptation.

The Four Pillars of Fitness

Regardless of age, gender, history, goals, or current fitness level, everyone will see optimal results when their regular exercise program includes a mix of the four most impacting factors of fitness: cardiovascular exercise, rest, flexibility, and strength. Whether you are a runner with a goal of beating your own 10-K record or a 50-year-old female exercising for the first time in 2 decades, balanced fitness will help you reach your goals faster.

As it pertains to the particulars (i.e., number of days, percentage of flexibility versus cardio, amount of rest, etc.), you'll make those decisions yourself, based on the goals you've set. However, I'm about to give you the best possible scenario, and you get to customize it to work for you. Once you understand each of these four components, you'll be able to choose the program

that is right for you, one that you will love!

You'll notice, however, that I devote less info here to explaining the type of strength training I think you should use. That's because I think it's so important that I devoted a whole section of the book to it. You'll hear me say this again and again because it's true. Strength training is the fountain of youth. If you aren't doing it now, it's about time you begin. I give you everything you need to get started in Part 2, 3 Circuits, One Bangin' Body! (see page 208). Between these two chapters, you'll have all the knowledge you need to accelerate your quest for a bangin' bod!

The First Pillar: Cardio

Whether you want to lose weight, maintain your weight, reduce stress, or just live longer, cardio is a must. It's nonnegotiable. Getting your heart rate up every day for a minimum of 30 minutes needs to be as routine as brushing your teeth.

The good news is you have plenty of choices for your cardio exercise. The best cardio workout is the one that you look forward to, the one that makes you want to push! Your soul-mate workout should be some form of cardio. I don't care if you're playing a round of speed golf or walking down the street pumping your arms like a crazy person, as long as you're enjoying it, you're breathing heavily, and your heart is pumping harder, I'm happy! Just about anything that gets your heart rate up for 30 minutes or more is fair game!

Specifically, you want to use a cardio workout that takes your intensity level up between 5 and 9 on a scale of 1 to 10. Lots of people talk about using heart rates and heart rate monitors or estimating the intensity of certain activities, but I have found that the RPE scale (see page 96) is so simple and so basic that anyone can use it to assess the effectiveness of a workout. I've modified it slightly, but I think you'll find it quite self-explanatory.

There are a bazillion different types of cardio workouts from which you can choose. I could write a 500-page book just on cardio workouts! But to summarize, I'll group cardio workouts in two categories and include a few examples:

Category 1: Impact

Low impact: Walking, some rock climbing, cycling, waterskiing, snowboarding, rowing, Pilates, yoga

High impact: Running, kickboxing, jumping rope, boxing, basketball, football, soccer

Category 2: Intensity

Moderate intensity: Walking, rock climbing, riding a bike, weight training, some yoga, and Pilates

Interval training: Competitive soccer, cycling, some aerobic fitness classes and DVDs

High-intensity interval training: Competitive basketball, competitive soccer, athletic drills, volleyball

Intensity is determined more by your effort than the workout you chose. I've seen plenty of people in the back of my Turbo Kick class, which is considered an intense workout, putting forth virtually no effort. That's why the best cardio workout is the one you like enough to actually

push yourself into those 7, 8, and 9 levels on the RPE chart!

To build a bangin' body, you want to have variety in the intensity, duration, and type of cardio you do. Regardless of the activity, you'll see improvements. But if you want a bangin' body, you'll see the best results when you get to a point that you committed to my 3-2-1 formula:

3 days of high-intensity or interval workouts of 30 minutes or more

2 days moderate-intensity, long-duration cardio (45 to 60 minutes)

1 day of moderate to low-intensity cardio activity for 30 minutes or more

The Second Pillar: Rest

When hungry eat, when tired sleep.
—Chinese proverb

There are mountains of research suggesting that Americans are overweight in large part because we are chronically sleep deprived (among other factors). Somewhere along the line, we've been brainwashed into thinking that rest or sleep is something lazy people do. This carries over into fitness, where many people say they are too tired to exercise. Those who work hard and miss the rest they so desperately need never allow their bodies to heal or to achieve adequate recovery.

Science teaches us that adequate hours and quality of sleep will help:

- Metabolize carbohydrates properly.

- Maintain leptin and growth hormones.

- Increase energy levels.

- Increase cognitive abilities.

- Maintain proper blood pressure and insulin resistance.

- Decrease anxiety and perceived stress.

- Repair muscle.

Most people fall off the exercise wagon after just a few weeks of effort. They fail to make adjustments in their sleeping patterns, and the result is a tired body and defeated resolve. Without enough sleep, it's difficult to do just about anything, let alone exercise and eat right.

It generally takes about 7 hours of quality sleep for most people to gain the reparations and benefits of sleep. People often lose sleep when they add exercise to the equation. This happens only when exercise is simply added to the existing busy schedule and no accommodations are made to scrape other activities off your plate!

Make an effort to measure and record your sleep hours and quality as carefully as you track your progress in any other area. Devices like the Bodybugg and Fitbit, worn while you sleep, can help you track and improve your sleep patterns.

MUSCLE REST

Your body needs adequate time to recuperate after exercise. The quicker the recovery, the quicker you'll see gains in strength and physical transformation. Strength and muscle gains (which translate into fat loss) increase during periods of rest. The amount of rest needed will vary from person to person based on your goals, your intensity, and your unique makeup.

Here are a few general guidelines to consider when planning rest:

- Moderate muscle soreness is normal.

- Intense muscle soreness means those muscle should not be "loaded" for a period of 24 hours of rest. That is not to say, however,

Rating of Perceived Exertion (RPE) Scale

1   Inactive—Virtually no change in heart rate.
2   Barely moving—Slight change in heart rate.
3   Moderate—I'm moving but could do this for hours.
4   Getting tough—But sustainable for long durations.
5   Tough—But I can still work and talk at the same time.
6   Even tougher—Sentences are turning into staggered words.
7   Very hard—Breathing hard, concentrating.
8   Very intense—Have to push myself and concentrate to maintain this level.
9   Superintense—A world outside this exercise simply doesn't exist.
10 Very, very hard—I can only go a few seconds at this level!

that you can't work the lactic acid and soreness out by doing something of moderate intensity.

- When weight training for strength, allow 24 hours of rest between muscle groups targeted in that day's workout.

- A day of rest after physically overloading your body is strongly encouraged. However, a brisk walk can be considered rest! There's a difference between elevating your heart rate and enjoying the mental benefits of moderate activity versus pushing yourself and taxing or loading your system.

Listen to your body, but don't be an excuse maker! Everyone needs rest. Your best progress will be made during periods of sleep and when you allow your body to repair itself. Here's my honest-to-goodness rule for rest: I do not schedule a day of rest for myself, I let "life" do that for me. In other words, I set out to get 7 days of exercise in per week, but at least once a week, or 2 days out of 10, something more important than my workout comes up. No problem! Instead of rigidly denying life's little surprises, I chalk them up to rest days. Granted, I will still find a way to get my heart rate up for a minimum of 30 minutes on those days (for the mental benefits), but it's not life and death.

The Third Pillar: Flexibility

Have you ever stood up after sitting for a prolonged period and felt the tightening and stiffness in your muscles? Then it's likely you need to improve your flexibility.

It's also likely that you know that. Yet flexibility is one of the most commonly neglected areas of fitness, perhaps because the progress is not visibly apparent. (Let's face it—when was the last time a beautiful girl walked by and you thought, "Man, she's got very flexible quadriceps"? Just doesn't happen.)

But improving flexibility does a body good. A flexible muscle has greater strength potential. Improved flexibility increases cardiovascular endurance and performance. With increased flexibility, you'll also move more comfortably, avoid injury, and whatever you do—from stooping to pick up a piece of paper to stretching to grab something off a tall shelf—will feel easier.

That said, you'll spend the smallest amount of time working on flexibility. That is not to diminish its importance but to help you prioritize the time you have to devote to fitness.

Your goal may involve dramatic gains in flexibility, but for most of us, flexibility objectives center around improving our function in everyday life. The easiest way to maintain your current level of flexibility is simply to stretch for 5 minutes after your cardio, while your muscles are warm and pliable.

That 5-minute postcardio stretch will help you maintain your flexibility. To actually improve it, you'll need to devote 1 to 2 days a week to flexibility training. It doesn't take much time, either. Simply tack an additional 20 to 30 minutes onto your postcardio or post-strength-training stretch and relax 1 to 2 days a week.

Improving your flexibility, and including flexibility exercises as part of your regular routine, might not get the scale to move as quickly as a run or eating the right foods, but it will give you an edge. Consider the benefits of improved flexibility:

- More energy and mobility
- More muscle strength and power
- Improved posture and balance
- Better athletic performance
- Reduced stiffness and joint pain
- Reduced muscle stress and chronic injury

The Fourth Pillar: Strength

Get excited! This is where it's at! This is where the kind of training you do can make all the difference in the world. Muscle is your fountain of youth! It's your secret weapon in the war against fat! It's your best friend who will make sure you burn more calories. (And that means you get to eat more! Yahoo!) Learn to love and appreciate muscle. Muscle is beautiful. Muscle is the most important component in building a bangin' body!

I'll give you the basics here, but you'll find the real, nitty-gritty deal begins on page 211.

MUSCLE FACT AND FICTION

A common misconception or fear that many people have, especially women, is that if they lift heavy weights, they will bulk up. Argggh!!! FALSE! I've got scientifically accurate news for you: Unless you're taking steroids, muscle will not bulk you up. Muscle leans you out.

Fat bulks you up.

Unfortunately, the idea that muscle will bulk you up is perpetuated by silly celebrities claiming they chiseled their tiny little bodies by lifting pink 3-pound baby weights or doing leg circles.

Strength-Training Facts

▶ **A body with more muscle tissue** burns more calories all day long, even when you aren't lifting a finger.

▶ **As you increase muscle composition through strength training,** you burn more calories when performing cardiovascular exercises.

▶ **Muscle provides shape.** Want a nice high booty? That takes muscle. Cardio doesn't "lift" body parts. The only tissue that really lifts and complements your shape is muscle.

▶ **Not all strength training is created equal.** Select a strength-training program scientifically proven to support the goals you have set for yourself.

▶ **For fat loss,** choose strength-building exercise, heavier weights, fewer reps.

▶ **For muscular endurance** sport-specific training, choose strength-training programs that promote endurance (lighter weights, greater reps, longer workouts).

Not. Sadly, once most celebrities leave the glare of Hollywood's harsh lights, we learn those frail frames are the result of deadly eating disorders. (Don't get me started.)

Let's talk birds and bees. Men and women are different. We have different hormones and biology. Aside from the obvious differences, in relation to women and weight training, the most important difference in body composition for women is the lower level of testosterone. This one difference inhibits the female body from producing muscle mass like our male counterparts.

Here's what that means in terms of muscle development for men and women. Simply stated, men build muscular size, which reduces body fat. That reduction of body fat results in bigger muscles and smaller waistlines. Sure, men put on weight all over, but primarily in their abdominal

Daily PUSH

1. Put together a workout plan for the week incorporating my suggested formula.

2. Research a strength-training DVD or class or find a personal trainer to help you begin building muscle ASAP!

NOTES

_____

_____

_____

_____

_____

_____

region. Whereas most women get chunky all over.

When women add muscle strength, they get smaller everywhere. Now in defense of women and weight lifting, this can be a key element in fat loss for women. Statistically speaking, women who lift weights to build strength (as opposed to endurance) will see a reduction in all measurements. Despite the gains in the strength, the female body burns fat as it builds muscle. That loss of fat just beneath the skin (aka *subcutaneous* fat) results in smaller measurements—everywhere!

DURATION AND FREQUENCY

I want you to aim for 6 days of exercise a week, 30 to 120 minutes a day, including multiple modes of fitness.

Approximately 60 percent of people who start exercise programs end up dropping out. To maximize the chances of success and adherence to the regimen, the specifics of the program—primarily, the frequency and duration of the workouts—must fit with the person's overall lifestyle. The best exercise program is tailored to meet specific needs and goals of a particular individual. What works for one person may not work well for another, so each person must determine what works best for her or him.

BE YOUR OWN TRAINER!

I've shared with you my honest evaluation of the exercise formula that research demonstrates will provide you with the very best results. Can you get a bangin' body by spending a negligible amount of time on flexibility or by creating your own hybrid program that looks nothing like what I've detailed? Sure. But why not use what we know works?

Become a student. Rather than simply learning proper form and technique, take your program a step further. Seek to understand more about how your body works and how one muscle affects the next. Learning about your body is like learning *why* it's important to put on sunscreen as opposed to just habitually applying it.

You're the right person for this job. You have a vested interest in your client! You have as much or more knowledge about your body and your goals than anyone you could hire. You are so much closer than you think. You have solid, scientifically proven information that will give you the edge. All you have to do is commit. Muscle is your fountain of youth, your secret weapon, and the key component to your bangin' body. Go get you some!

DAY 14
DESTINATION FIXATION

To Win the Race, Focus on Your Finish

Today we'll work work on the habit of focusing our minds on what we want to have happen as opposed to the 90 bazillion things that could go wrong.

Destination fixation is a term I heard when I was a kid learning to ride a motorcycle. My dad has loved motorcycles his whole life. He's been a bike mechanic and a bike salesman, and now that he has the means, he's a collector. He had me on a motorcycle before my 5th birthday, riding on trails and racing the boys. One of the first things Dad taught me was: "Where you look is where you go."

When I was very young, my dad entered me in motocross events called trials. These are very different from traditional motocross races, where the first person who crosses the finish line wins. In trials, a specialized, rugged outdoor terrain is designed to test the riders' ability to focus despite myriad obstacles. The races are often held in wooded areas with mud, sand, dirt, debris, logs, and intentionally treacherous terrain. Your success in trials is judged by the number of times you need to put a foot down to catch your balance, your bike rolls backward, or you are forced off your bike by an obstacle.

Trials training requires balance, patience, and focus on where you're headed. If you look at a tree stump, you will run into the tree stump and probably need to put your foot down. I learned, however, that if I looked out in front of me, in the direction I was headed, I would roll right over the tree stump as if it were an inconsequential bump in the road.

If you've tried snowboarding or if you learned to ride a bike, you have experienced destination fixation. The general concept: *Look at it, run into it.*

You look at the curb. You think, "I don't want to run into the curb. I hope I don't run into that curb. That curb is getting closer. I can't look away. Oh no!!! I'm hitting the curb!" And sure enough, you fixate yourself into a crash.

If at the moment you glanced at the curb, you then immediately fixed your eyes back on your destination, you would have been able to pull out of the collision. Instead of looking at obstacles, instead of focusing on what you *don't* want to do, fixate on your finish line. Fix your gaze on where it is you want to end up!

Today we'll explore how this concept applies to anything you've done that involves a journey or final destination. It's time to work on catching ourselves when we start to focus on anything *other* than our "destination"—the final outcome or the positive end result of our goals. By rejecting negative thoughts, you will in turn avoid focusing on your obstacles and instead redirect your concentration to the finish line.

Watch Out for That Tree!

I bet you've experienced something similar to this: I grew up a skier. In fact, I cursed those crazy kids on snowboards. "They're obnoxious and rude and they're messing up my run!" I thought. With 35 years on skis, I vowed to never venture to the dark side.

But when Bret and I had kids and watched our little skiers looking longingly at the cool kids on snowboards, I realized it was time for us all to give it a try.

Fast-forward 5 years and now I'm a total Betty (slang for a chick who snowboards). It has become a soul-mate workout! It is by far our favorite activity as a family. It's killer fun for everyone to race down the mountain, testing our physical limits, getting a great workout, rocking out to music on headsets that also allow you to hear what's going on around you, and loving every minute of it together. I can't say enough great things about having a family sport.

Last year Bret bought me a new snowboard for Christmas. It was bigger, faster, and a lot scarier than the snowboard I used the previous season. I was grateful for the gift but a little freaked out by the challenge.

My debut on this new board felt like my first day ever on the mountain. I was anxious and stiff. The whole family waited for me while I nervously navigated each turn as if the powder had transformed into a sheet of ice. To make matters worse, I kept running into things, including some very unhappy skiers, the out-of-bounds markers, rocks, giant moguls, and just about everything else that was to be avoided. If it was going to run me off course, I looked at it, freaked out that I was going to hit it, and then promptly did.

Finally Bret crinkled down his eyebrows like he does and said, "What's going on with you? You're such a great rider, and this board is not that much different. Why are you running into everything?"

Destination fixation! That was it! That was my problem and my solution.

So the next day when we hit the slopes, I said, "No more looking at obstacles. No one wait for me!" I told the kids, "Fly ahead and I'll keep my eyes on you." I focused only on where it was they were headed. I looked off into the distance and kept my eyes on the end of the trail or the chairlift at the bottom of the hill. As soon as I did, I relaxed and enjoyed the ride. I actually fell in love with my new board.

Focus on Your Finish

What I'm trying to say is this: Stop worrying and obsessing about the person you think might be holding you back or the skill you don't yet have or all of the other things you could possibly run into. Because if you're fixating on them, you will indeed run into them. Start fixating on your destination—your goal, the end product. Don't let those other things distract you.

Learning to focus on your outcome is a habit. As you learn this habit, you may need to start with baby steps. Begin by thinking about the one thing this week you need to accomplish.

Let's say that one thing is to create a 3,500-calorie deficit to be on track to lose another pound. Yet, every time you think about your goal, you reflect on how difficult it's going to be to eat healthy at Lisa's baby shower on Sunday, or you ponder all the temptations of homemade desserts that loom in the office lunchroom and how your husband planned a pizza party for the kids.

Your first step is to catch yourself and realize those thoughts represent the curb you don't want to hit. Instead, focus on your finish line. Those negative thoughts are obstacles for the former you but inconsequential bumps in the road for the new, highly focused you.

Make your final destination your only option by focusing on the positive tools you have in place.

Self-Correct Your Focus

Try this suggestion out yourself. The next social event you attend where you have no clue who half the people are, or what they might be thinking about you, avoid accessorizing with anxiety. Self-doubt doesn't look good on anyone! Not helping.

Picture yourself being loved and admired by everyone you meet. Assume that all in attendance have heard great things about you. Assume in advance that people will like you exactly the way you are. Tell yourself that a cold or less-than-interested greeting is simply the other person's nervousness or anxiety. Assume that people already think the world of you, so there's no need to prove or doubt yourself. Make it your goal to want to know more about each person you encounter. Make it a game, a challenge to meet as many people as possible and make *them* feel comfortable.

Instead of responding to the urge to tell others about yourself and your accomplishments and then worry endlessly about their opinion of you, focus on *them*. Make it your goal to listen to the people you meet. Collect the life stories of others. Ask open-ended questions. Listen. Digest. Be present.

As with any skill or habit, practice makes perfect. Before long, you'll be much quicker to catch yourself fixating on an obstacle or fear. You'll get in the habit of redirecting your own focus and reframing your concentration.

Create a No-Crash Zone

If you truly believe that success is your only option, than success will be your destination. If you believe that bad luck, deceitful people, and a predetermined gene for obesity are your obstacles, then guess where you're headed? Give

Daily**PUSH**

1. List any idea, person, skill, or circumstance that you have perceived to be a possible obstacle on your journey toward achieving your Push goal and your health goal.

2. Now cross that item off. Physically take a pen and draw a line or an *X* through that perceived obstacle.

3. List one positive thing you will focus on when you think of reaching your Push or your health goal.

4. Now use the item you listed in step 1 as your trigger. Each time you picture that perceived obstacle, you will be reminded to replace that thought with your positive focus listed in step 3.

EXAMPLE:

Perceived obstacle: "I don't have money for a gym membership."

Positive: My mentor lost 100 pounds—without a gym membership.

Trigger response: When I begin to worry that I won't reach my goal because I don't have a gym membership, I will immediately replace that thought with the image of my inspiration: Getting ripped and fit at home!

energy to your roadblocks, and they'll flip you off course. When you focus on the person or the limitations you believe you have, you will gain nothing more than an ulcer.

Allow only your destination to dominate your thinking. Paint a picture in your mind of what your goal looks like once achieved. Imagine how you'd feel. Embrace the excitement of crossing the finish line as if you've just done so.

Only you can chart and keep yourself on course. You control your destiny. Where you look is where you will go. What you want to see is what will appear in front of you. What you focus on becomes your reality. Expect the best of people. Avoid looking straight down, behind you, or at the many obstacles that if given your attention will force you to put your foot down. Focus a little farther down the road, in the direc-tion of your destination. Expect that you will succeed. Expect that every goal on your list will be achieved.

Fixate on Your Goals

Learning to focus on the positive is your new habit. It's not technical or a part of your genetic makeup. You're not naturally a glass-half-full kinda person. You've just allowed yourself to create a negative habit. All bad habits can be broken, and all good habits can be learned. Fixate on your goals. Learning this habit will take self-awareness and persistence, but the more you do it, the easier it becomes. Before long, you'll be rushing toward your destination at an exhilarating speed!

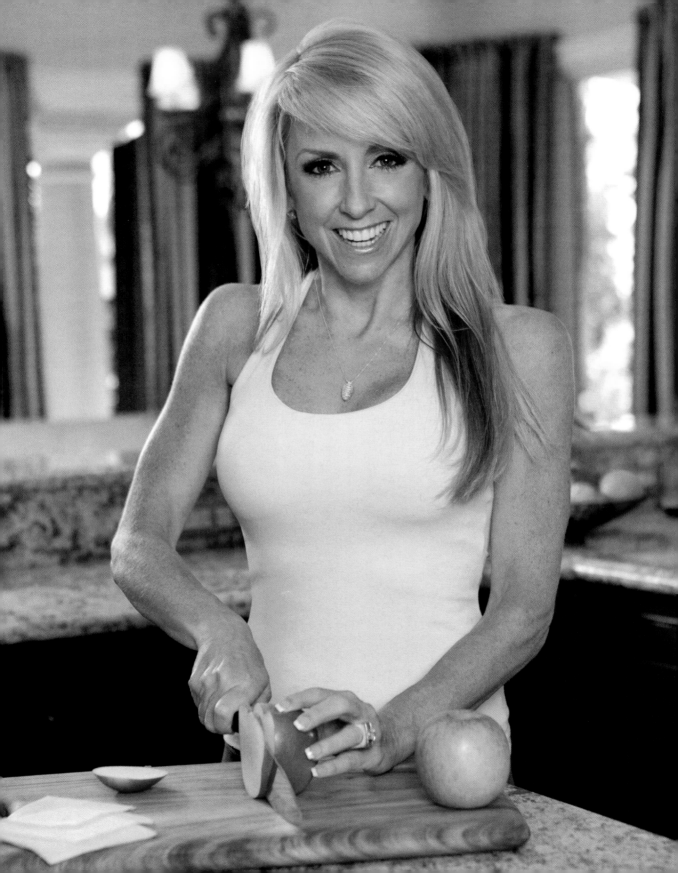

KITCHEN MAKEOVER

It's All in the Presentation

Surprise! Today you're getting a kitchen makeover! Sorry, that cute Ty Pennington, host of *Extreme Home Makeover,* with his little puka shell necklace, will not be showing up at your door. But then again, your makeover won't be that extreme. In fact, this won't take long at all!

Today I'll share with you how to reorganize your kitchen, pantry, and fridge so that success is not just simple and convenient but visually enticing!

Your kitchen makeover starts with making it convenient and easy to eat healthfully. Creating a healthy kitchen boils down to the following:

1. Gathering the proper tools and ensuring easy access to them.

2. Repackaging bulk items into single servings.

3. Placing fruits, vegetables, and healthful foods and snacks at eye level.

Right Tools in the Right Place

Each tool that you use on a daily and perhaps even mealtime basis should be kept close to the area where you prep your food. I suggest having the following all in one drawer, plastic container, or cupboard for quick and easy access:

- Paring knife
- Vegetable peeler
- Measuring cup

- Food scale
- Snack-size plastic bags
- Plastic 1-cup-size reusable containers

Repackage Your Food

Warning: Open bags can lead to saddlebags. You and I both know we are going to keep reaching into that bag of snacks or treats and eat well beyond an individual portion. Here's what I do: Repackage bulk snacks—say, raw almonds—into appropriate serving sizes. When you come home from food shopping, take the time to divvy up food by serving size. If you have small humans in your home, this is a wonderful way for them to earn their keep and help mom!

Use small plastic bags or reusable plastic storage containers to organize your food into the right portions. For example, my kids love whole wheat pretzel rods. A portion size for this snack is 10 sticks (they're about the size of a child's pinky finger). I fill up little bags, throw them in the pantry at eye level, and make it simple for grab-and-go snacking.

A recent Cornell University study found that we consume 90 percent of our food mindlessly. We eat simply because it has been placed in front of us (or because we've placed it in front of ourselves). It's time to get conscious about what—and how much—we consume.

Children in Africa Do Not Want Last Year's Halloween Candy

Most of us are terrified to throw even the junkiest of junk food away. Perhaps it's because in the back of our minds we can hear our mothers reminding us that children in a third-world country will go to bed tonight hungry. That's true. So send your financial contributions if you want to help, but that box of Ho Hos . . . they don't need 'em.

Dump or donate anything that a well-tuned athlete wouldn't eat. If that box of Lucky Charms for your kids is constantly calling your name, ditch it. Stepping into your kitchen shouldn't be an anxiety-producing situation. Make it easier on yourself to make healthy choices by eliminating the temptation of poor choices.

Tip: Unless you live alone, you might want to dump the junk a few items a day rather than all at once. The more clandestine you can be about this operation, the less friction you'll encounter from the troops! One of the kids asked me where the sugar-filled breakfast bars had gone, about 2 years after I had thrown out what was left and vowed to stop bringing them home from the market. (If you don't mention it, they'll probably never notice!)

Merchandise Your Food

Food marketers and stylists play into our impulsive choices by paying millions of dollars every year to have name-brand products placed on the right shelf at the right level. Why do you think all the sugary cereals are placed at your chest level on the shelves of your grocery? It's because that happens to be the eye line of a child sitting in a shopping cart. Clever!

Let's talk placement! You too can use this same technique to your advantage in your own fridge and pantry.

Refrigerator Makeover

When we stand in front of the fridge, we tend to grab whatever food takes the least amount of time to prepare and that "looks good." The healthy stuff, like fresh produce, we hide in a drawer that's difficult to get to and even easier to forget! I think they call that drawer the crisper, but they should really call it the rotter. By the time you remember there's something down there, it's rotten! Then the thought of the money we've wasted deters us from buying more.

Until refrigerator manufacturers figure this out, we have to take matters into our own hands and be smart about how we showcase our food in our own fridges.

UNLOAD, WASH, DISPLAY As you unload your groceries, clean and display your fruit in clear plastic containers or bowls. Place berries and raw veggies at eye level. Use a fully organic fruit/veggie spray like Eat Cleaner to naturally prolong the life of your produce and to strip away pesticides, bacteria, and waxes. An all-natural produce spray brings out the natural colors of your fruits and veggies, making them even more enticing. Cut raw vegetables, or heck, you don't have to impress me, buy them precut! But then display them for easy snacking.

Arrange your fat-free Greek yogurt near the berries and veggies. Store low-fat cottage cheese nearby as well. Place healthy whole foods at eye level near the front of the shelf.

When you're building muscle, hard-cooked egg whites are a great source of lean protein, and they're easy to prep so they're ready to go! Boil a dozen eggs on Sunday night, then peel and place them in a large plastic storage bag! Now, all you have to do is remove the yolk (or not), dice up your egg whites, dump some salsa in there, and *BAM!*

Other fast protein sources to be stored at eye level include prepackaged tuna packets. Though they store well in the pantry, I keep them in the refrigerator. Who wants a warm tuna sandwich? They come in different flavors such as herb and lemon that are so tasty you don't even need to doll 'em up!

Now when you find yourself staring mindlessly into your fridge, you'll see the stuff you *should* be eating! It's washed, cut, enticing, and ready to go.

REPLACE THIS WITH THAT Look in your refrigerator for regular staples. Now, do some soul searching and ask yourself if you're willing to try a healthier alternative. Do you make the kids PB&J every week? Would they notice if you picked up a sugar-free or low-sugar jar of jam or jelly? If you don't say anything . . . probably not!

I *l-o-v-e* cheese. But, instead of buying a brick of it, I stock up on individually packaged fat-free-milk string cheese. They are portion controlled and appropriately sized. I don't have to take the time to look at the packaging to figure out how many ounces is a single serving.

What about trying lower-sugar or organic versions of many of your regular condiments? Ketchup, salad dressings, mayo, and butter are common staples of the fridge door. Look for healthier versions. For example, try spray butter at zero calories a spritz.

I know some of the food police will freak out at the mere mention of spray butter, but what's most important is that we start making small changes. Where can you make some healthy substitutions? Add those items to your grocery

Daily PUSH

1. Remove high-fat, high-sugar temptations from the kitchen.

2. Survey the refrigerator for frequently consumed foods that can be swapped out by lower fat and reduced-calorie alternatives.

3. Stock up on small plastic food bags, snack containers, and clear plastic fruit bowls for display.

4. Arrange prep tools in an easy-to-reach place. The fewer steps, the better!

5. Spring-clean your fridge! Make room for the fresh stuff.

6. Divide snacks into individual servings and arrange front and center in the pantry.

NOTES

_____

_____

_____

_____

list. Not sure which brand or version is the better choice? Apps like Fooducate allow you to scan the bar codes of two products and do a side-by-side comparison. Each item is given a grade based on its nutritional content, which makes it convenient for quick decisions. Surprisingly, spray butter doesn't score that poorly!

Pantry or Cupboard Makeover

Most of the healthiest foods will be perishable and stored in the refrigerator. Period. Once you have that in order, it's time to tackle your cupboards and/or pantry.

First, let's figure out why you would go to the pantry instead of your fridge. Well, we often go to the cupboard when we want carbs, something fast, something crunchy, something sweet. That's fine. But let's create healthier temptations. `DISPLAY` The pantry and cupboard make it easy to place food so that it's readily available. Those foods that are lower on the good-for-you hierarchy can go on the hard-to-reach, where-did-I-put-that-stepstool shelves!

I use the eye- and chest-level shelves (the most coveted shelves in your grocery stores) to place healthiest nonperishable items. Nothing bought in bulk ever stays in its original container. I open, repackage, and display these items in inexpensive containers, like wicker baskets or square plastic storage bins. It keeps things organized and makes choosing healthy so dummy-proof that the foods almost jump into my hand.

So here's what you'll find on my "expensive real estate" shelves:

- Packets of raw nuts
- Individual packets of protein cereal
- Instant oatmeal (again, out of the box and into a storage container)
- High-quality protein bars
- Dried fruit
- Wasa crackers
- Protein powders
- Instant sugar-free cocoa
- Whole grain cereal
- Canned soups/beans
- Instant precooked brown rice
- Bags of plain microwave popcorn

Will you be able to find cake mix, 100-calorie packs of cookies, or tortilla chips in my pantry? Probably, but you'll have to move a few things around or get up on a ladder to find them. Outta sight—outta mind! `ANOTHER GROCER'S SECRET` Put things where people know to look for them. I basically stock the same stuff all the time. I maintain a list and check off what I need. But there is no mystery. No one is opening the pantry and expecting a sudden influx of cookies or chips.

Boring? Yes! *Intentionally* boring. You see, if you never knew what you might get when you opened the pantry, you'd go there first. I don't want my family to eat from the pantry. The pantry is where emergency foods live. Let's face it, with few exceptions, just about everything in your pantry is processed. The healthy stuff is in the fridge! Pretty sneaky, sis!

DAY 16

Know Your
NUMBERS

*Success Is Predictable
When You Know the Formula!*

Scary fact: If you consume just 100 calories more than you need a day, you may very well gain as much as 10 pounds in a year. Yup—100 extra calories a *day* equals 10 pounds a *year*. Crazy, I know! That's why you have to "know your numbers." They include your basal metabolic rate (BMR), your body-fat percentage, and your daily calorie intake (DCI). Knowing your numbers is the key to not just losing weight but *maintaining that weight loss*.

So today's a big day for you. You'll learn why calories count (still, always, and forever) and why, if you have a history of crash dieting, you've probably diminished your body's ability to metabolize calories. Finally, you'll learn to calculate those numbers (and they're as unique as you are!).

Armed with this knowledge, you'll be able to get off the diet roller coaster for good. Yes, there's some math involved. But if you do it—and yes, you can use a calculator—there's no question about it: Losing weight will become a once-and-done deal. Success is like a combination lock; once you know the numbers, cracking the safe is easy.

The Ultimate No-Limits Spending Spree Is Yours!

Wouldn't that be awesome? No-limits spending is a dream scenario, far removed from the realities of our financial situations. It would be nice, but in the real world we must know the amount we have available to spend *before* we spend it. Even if math isn't our strong suit, as adults we have no choice but to do the math. (Are you getting an idea where I'm heading with this?)

Calories. Yup! You guessed it. There are many variables to weight loss, but the basic mathematical truth is that to lose a pound, you must create a deficit of 3,500 calories regardless of your metabolism, race, gender, or creed.

"Why count calories? Who wants to bother with numbers and points?" That's the marketing tactic of many diet experts and weight-loss infomercials. Knowing your numbers and keeping track of calories sound arduous and mundane. It takes effort. To suggest it's not necessary certainly appeals to masses of people who are looking for a shortcut.

When I hear other health professionals suggesting that you shouldn't worry about the balance of calories in versus calories out but rather eat clean and follow your hunger instincts, well, I really just want to pinch their heads off. That's like a millionaire suggesting that instead of worrying about what's in your bank account, just listen to your shopping instincts and buy high-quality goods.

Uh, *hello* . . . Earth to super-ripped, genetically gifted lean person who exercises every day . . . that's not going to work for the rest of the population.

Advising the average person to not concern herself with calories but instead to pay attention to hunger triggers and eating foods rich in nutrients—well, it's a wonderful concept. I also love the thought of unicorns jumping over cotton candy rainbows. I'm even considering taking up basketball to see if it makes me taller. Come on already! Suggesting that someone who struggles with his weight does not need to think about calories is just ludicrous. It really is as risky as suggesting you not look at price tags the next time you're in the market for a car.

Sorry to disappoint, but it is not possible to achieve six-pack abs by sitting on the couch wearing a special blue belt. Pull your head out of the sand, get real, and know your numbers. Your weight loss and body transformation will happen due to a series of steps that result in a shift in these numbers.

Numbers are significant. They tell us what we can or cannot afford. Numbers tell us how hard we need to work. Numbers help us keep score. Numbers tell us when we are winning. Numbers tell us when we have done enough and can enjoy the fruits of our labor.

Numbers matter!

To be fit and healthy for life, you must ascertain the number of calories required to strike a balance between what you need and how much you should cut back without creating a metabolic slowdown.

Calorie counting is just one element of knowing your numbers. True, not all calories are created equal, but that doesn't give us an excuse not to monitor them. Knowing your numbers includes knowing what you burn. Balancing calories in versus calories out might not sound like a party, but neither is balancing your checkbook. Both are necessary.

But here's the thing. While it's true that it takes a 3,500-calorie deficit to lose a pound, losing weight is *way* more than eating fewer calories and exercising.

Approaching 40, Fat, and I've Tried That

Calories count. But they're only one part of the weight-loss equation. The single most important thing you can do to *maintain* weight loss is *increase the speed of your metabolism.*

Maybe you know what I'm talking about, especially if you're over 30, approaching 40, or over 50 and frustrated. You gain weight by simply looking at the menu. Perhaps for the first time, you found yourself cutting back, dieting, and on the hunt for anything with stretch! (Even PajamaJeans caught your eye!)

By the time you hit 40, the fight is on in full force! Back fat and muffin tops are just something you learn to, *ahem,* fashionably conceal. Depression over your weight and the constant struggle to lose it has become the bane of your everyday life. Fat has settled into places you never had it before, and to lose 5 pounds takes total deprivation. Your

metabolism feels like it's crawling, and this whole numbers thing is just not adding up! It must be you. You must have a defective metabolism, some rare bloating disease. You curse your dryer for shrinking your clothes (even the ones you hang-dry) and resort to the only thing that has ever worked for you in the past: You cut calories. And cut calories. And cut some more.

How's that working out for you? It's not. In fact, it's the worst thing you can do. Consuming fewer calories than your BMR requirements is perhaps the single greatest reason why the diet industry is a multibillion-dollar giant. And it's the reason so many people end up destroying their metabolisms. Because they focus only on the 3,500-calorie deficit and work to create a dramatic deficit for as long as they can, the consequences of this approach, ironically, are weight gain, muscle loss, stored fat, and a metabolism only a turtle could appreciate.

All research points to the fact that if you eat too few calories, your body—the absolute most advanced machine on the planet—will slow your metabolism. To protect you from starvation, your ultrasmart machine-body will retain fat and slow your resting metabolic rate.

What's particularly tempting about crash diets and extreme calorie restrictions is that initially you do lose weight. How exciting is that?!? So you keep cutting back and your weight loss continues for a while. The first couple of days, the weight seems to fall off, and then your progress begins to slow. When you do ultimately have a "slip," you're mortified by how quickly the scale creeps back up.

You've probably spent enough time beating yourself up and trying to make sense of your inability to lose weight. You're not alone. It truly is an epidemic. You've been told that if you burn more than you consume, you'll lose weight. And guess what? It does work . . . for a while. But your body is a very intelligent machine.

Before long, your weight loss slows. As you continue to restrict calories and move more, the scale seems to be playing an evil joke on you. You're barely eating, you're exercising like a maniac, and you haven't had a piece of bread since 1999. You've gone organic, fat free, gluten free; eaten according to your body type; and done everything you've been told to do. You look in the mirror, grab a handful of spare tire, and scream, "So *WHY AM I SO FAT*?"

What did I tell you? You gotta know your numbers!

Your Personal Numbers

Weight loss is not magic. To a great extent, it's accounting. So if you're one of those people who have no idea how much money they have in the bank, or if you so despise math that you look the other way and sing "la la la la la," it's time to take your fingers out of your ears, sit up straight, and take some notes.

Your personal numbers begin with the humble calorie, a unit of energy. We get calories from the food we consume. *Metabolism* is the process by which your body converts food to energy. During this process, the calories in food combine with oxygen to release the energy your body needs to function.

When I say "your numbers," I'm referring to the following:

BMR (BASAL METABOLIC RATE) The number of calories you burn *in total*, including any and all exercise and the calories you need to sustain life. (You *do* burn calories when you're sleeping or loafing on the couch—your body needs energy to breathe, circulate blood, make and repair cells, and other important stuff.)

Your BMR is determined by several factors, including:

- **Gender.** Men typically have less body fat and more muscle than women of the same age and weight. Yup—men burn more calories. Totally unfair.

- **Age.** With every birthday, you tend to lose muscle and gain fat, which also slows down calorie burning. Also totally unfair.

- **Body size and composition.** If you're large, or have lots of muscle (remember this!), you'll burn more calories, even when you're slacking.

DCI (DAILY CALORIE INTAKE) You'll learn it today, and it's important. At any given moment, I can tell you within about 50 calories my DCI for that day. I also know my calorie burn for the same 24-hour period within a 10 percent margin of error. I'm not obsessed about it at all. Many days, I consume more than I burn, and there are just as many days that I burn more than I consume. That's how I strike a balance and maintain my weight.

These numbers don't solely work for me. If you're a carbon-based life-form, they'll work for you, too. And if anyone knows what I'm talking about, it's one of my clients, Cheryl.

Cheryl's Story

"I swear to you I'm eating less than a 2-year-old!" That's what Cheryl, 45, told me the first day we met. She'd been dieting off and off—mostly on—for 10 years. But although she had moderate success, the weight always came back.

In the past 2 years, despite her best efforts to lose weight, she had only gained it. Now 50 pounds overweight, she was also struggling with the emotional toll of a divorce, raising two boys on her own, and the recent death of her father. She came to me desperate for a solution.

I'm embarrassed to admit that I thought to myself, "Yeah, right, lady. If you were eating as well as you say, you wouldn't be 50 pounds overweight." I assumed that dieting had slowed her metabolism and that the stress wasn't helping much.

Though I could have tested her body fat and BMR with my own body-fat calipers or a digital device, I wanted unquestioned accuracy. So I arranged to have her BMR tested hydrostatically. (Hydrostatic body-fat testing is the industry gold standard.)

According to Cheryl's food journal, she was eating between 800 and 900 calories a day—near starvation for a woman of 5 foot 2 inches. I admit, I was skeptical. I assumed our findings would support my assumptions—that she was consuming wa-a-a-ay more calories than that—and the testing would serve as Cheryl's wakeup call to be more forthcoming with her food journal.

But what I was about to find out blew my mind.

According to the most accurate body-fat test-ing method available today, her resting metabolic rate was *732 calories*.

Whaaaaaaaaat?!

That meant if this sweet, 45-year-old woman decided to eat 1,000 calories a day, she would be on pace to gain more than 20 pounds a year, which was exactly what she was doing. I don't know if you've ever tried to follow a 1,000-calorie-a-day diet, but I assure you spending time in a POW camp would be more nutritionally satisfying.

Now that Cheryl knew her numbers, we could develop a plan that made sense, numerically. We could add food to her plate, muscle to her body, and create a hostile environment for fat!

Our first order of business: to radically *increase* Cheryl's BMR. To do it, she needed to change her body's ratio of fat to lean tissue. In other words, she needed to build muscle.

To build muscle, she had to do two things. The first: Begin a strength-training program. Cheryl had never, and I mean never, exercised in her whole life and, quite frankly, was none too excited to start.

Until she saw her numbers change *the very first day*. Exercise increased Cheryl's numbers in two areas: BMR and daily calorie burn. Immediately—as in day one of exercise—she was burning in the range of 1,000 to 1,200 calories per day!

The second thing Cheryl had to do was eat more. Had she stayed in starvation mode while trying to build muscle, her body would continue to store fat. To increase her BMR, I had her began to consume between 1,000 and 1,200 calories daily—the same number she now burned per day.

Cheryl also started following my approach to food selection (which some people call a diet). She began eating more slow-to-metabolize foods dense in nutrients, complex carbohydrates, and lean proteins, plus fruit, which is naturally filling due to its high content of fiber.

Eating more completely freaked Cheryl out. "I can't eat all this food," she said every time we met. "I'm so full. I've never eaten this much. I know I'm going to gain weight. I'm afraid to get on the scale."

Thirty days after Cheryl started strength training and her new way of eating, we had her body fat and BMR measured again. She'd reduced her body fat *by almost 20 percent.*

We tested again on Day 60 and once more on Day 90. Within 3 months, she increased her BMR to almost 1,300 calories and reduced her body fat *by over 50 percent.*

Astonishing to Cheryl, predictable to me. It'll happen for you, too—and when it does, I won't be surprised, either.

How Do Your Numbers Add Up?

Here's what your numbers mean. To lose a pound, you need to create a deficit of 3,500 calories. To gain a pound, you eat 3,500 calories more than you expend. To know if you've gone over your daily calorie requirements, you need to know what you burn. Most people use only their weight and age to determine their average calorie expenditure, when actually your body fat has a dramatic impact on the amount of calories you burn. So, let's say that you determine your body-fat percentage, and that allows you to create a very accurate assessment of your BMR as around 2,000 calories. Now we'll add a workout to that equation and you're burning around 2,600 calories in a 24-hour period.

To lose a pound a week, you'll have to consume an average of 2,100—and that's assuming you're exercising every day. Instead, let's say you will exercise 5 days a week. Well, that would mean you're burning roughly 17,000 calories a week. Now take 17,000 and subtract the 1 pound of weight you'd like to lose . . . that's 17,000-3,500 = 13,500 calories you can consume. This means, on average, your diet should be around 1,900 calories a day—and that's of course assuming you're working out hard and being really honest about what you're eating.

But what if you want to lose 2 pounds per week? Then you would take your 17,000 (total average calories burned for a 7-day period) and subtract 7,000 calories, resulting in 10,000 calories you can take in per week. Therefore, to lose 2 pounds per week, you'd need to consume around 1,430 calories per day.

Is there more to it? Of course. As you continue to exercise and add muscle to the equation, you'll increase your BMR. You may find yourself becoming more active in general, which will also raise your BMR. You may find a workout that allows you to burn more calories. Or you might have a week when you can't exercise at all, in which case you'll need to adjust your calorie intake. But all of this hinges on your knowing your numbers.

Now we're at the nitty-gritty: determining your BMR, body fat, and DCI. You can do this several different ways, listed in order of accuracy. *Here's a success tip. This might look like a lot. It's not. I just want you to see all the practical options available to you. As you read through these options, highlight the one(s) that will work for you.*

1. Body fat and BMR.

> **a.** Schedule a "dunk" with a local provider of hydrostatic body-fat testing. During the test, you are submerged in water while your underwater weight is recorded. Many universities offer hydrostatic weight tests, but several companies offer testing for the public. Body Fat Test (www.bodyfattest.com) provides a mobile hydrostatic body composition testing service in a variety of locations throughout the United States. FinessWave (www.getdunked.com) offers underwater weighing in locations in several states nationwide.

> **b.** Use a reputable calorie-recording device such as the Bodybugg or Fitbit. You wear these high-tech gadgets, which keep an accurate daily record of calories consumed versus burned. They run from $100 (Fitbit) to $300 (Bodybugg), but if you can afford it, they're worth the investment! To check out these devices, log on to www.fitbit.com or www.bodybugg.com.

> **c.** If you like math, you can calculate an estimate of your BMR using the formula below. If you don't like math, you'll want to use a calculator.

If you're a woman:
BMR = 655 + (4.35 x weight in pounds) + (4.7 x height in inches) - (4.7 x age in years)
   So if you're a 48-year-old, 130-pound woman who is 5 foot 2 inches, your equation would look like this:
BMR = 655 + (565.5) + (291.4) - (225.6) = 1,286

If you're a man:
BMR = 66 + (6.23 x weight in pounds) + (12.7 x height in inches) - (6.8 x age in years)

d. Finally, if you don't have a calculator on hand, you can visit one of several free Web sites that offer BMR calculators. Most also include formulas for you to estimate your body-fat percentage. Remember that these are estimates. Always err on the side of caution and assume you're not burning as much as they say you do. That way you'll be on the safe side. These sites include:

▶ Discovery Health (http://health.discovery.com/centers/heart/basal/basal.html)

▶ InternetFitness.com (www.internetfitness.com/calculators/bmr.htm)

▶ SparkPeople (www.sparkpeople.com)

2. DCI. Record your daily calorie intake with exacting accuracy (at least in the beginning to get a baseline). That means tracking those extra few bites of leftover mac and cheese from your kid's plate, the piece of candy you snuck out of your co-worker's candy dish, everything that passes your lips. (Don't cheat. Don't leave things off your list. Lying to yourself will only hurt you in the long run.)

3. Take your BMR and add the calories you burn each day based on physical exercise and additional activity. You can do this in the following ways, as listed below in order of accuracy:

a. A calorie monitoring device like the Bodybugg or Fitbit

b. Free exercise calorie calculator (listed above in subsection 1d)

c. By using the readout listed on many cardio machines (This estimate is often the least accurate, as it provides an estimate of calories burned based on the average height-and-weight male.)

4. For a down and dirty estimate of your total daily needs and expenditure, finish this equation:

Total calories you consumed in the last 24 hours: _____

(Minus)

Total calories you burned in the last 24 hours: _____

▶ **Deficit/surplus created:** _____

DAY 17

The **PUSH PLAN**

A Tiered Approach to Eating

To accomplish 10 crazy cool things in the next year, you need *all* areas of your life in alignment. Picture yourself driving down the road toward your Push goal. Your well-tuned vehicle carries prize cargo in every seat. You've downloaded your map, checked the tire pressure, and ensured that the wheels are aligned, the oil changed, and the interior detailed. *And* you made the perfect playlist for your journey. Knowing the significance of your destination (hint, hint: look at your list of 10 if you need a reminder), you know that it's critical to use the highest-grade fuel. The right fuel will get you there—quickly.

Today you discover a way to eat for the rest of your life that gives you optimal results, sustained health, and something to look forward to at each meal.

I'd like to share with you my own simple three-tiered approach to nutrition that mirrors our traffic light system. The colors green, yellow, and red are used as a simple-to-understand,

easy-to-identify universal rating system that allows me to make split-second decisions. Look, we've probably all run a red light, heart racing and knuckles clenched around the wheel, and lived to tell the tale. Each of us has watched a light turn yellow and thought, "Oh, it just turned. I'm fine." Or "Shoot. I'm really pushing it. This could turn red any moment." But most of the time, we obey the rules of the road. Green means go. Red means stop. Yellow means apply the brakes. Our experience on the road, our love for life, our respect for the people we love dictates our decision each time we approach a traffic light. Now you can begin to apply the same approach to food.

"Tiered eating" is designed to help you find the "best" way to eat—that is, the diet that fits with your lifestyle, tastes, and priorities. It allows you to eat without guilt and enjoy the life you want—and isn't that the whole point?

This approach to eating doesn't end after 30 days or when you hit your "target weight." This plan is for life. Can you imagine Bill Gates thinking that he would learn the habits of successful entrepreneurs before him, follow them until he made his first million, then go back to his old ways? Hell no! Once you get good at being a healthy person, once you enjoy success because it's your own creation, the only thing that changes is that you want to keep getting better!

Your Life, Your Choices

When I was a child, my parents rarely told us kids what we *had* to do. They guided us. They offered their opinions, explained the possible outcomes or consequences, and then charged us with the responsibility of making the right decision. When in the ninth grade I announced I'd like to dye part of my hair pink, shave one side with stripes, and have a tail to braid down the side (circa 1984 Cyndi Lauper), they explained

that in such a small town I could expect to be teased and talked about. They cautioned me that certain parents might make assumptions about my character or go as far as to not allow their daughters to hang out with me. My mom thought the idea was "wicked cool" but warned me that my volleyball coach might not look favorably on a punk-rock hairdo. *Okay, I'll think about it.*

Monday afternoon, I showed up to practice with my "totally awesome" hair. By halftime of Thursday night's game, I was already calculating how long it would take to grow it out. The experience, however, gave me the confidence to make my own decisions, knowing that if I made a wrong one, I would have to live with it. My parents gave me the information and offered their advice, but ultimately the choice was *usually* left up to me. "You'll make an appropriate decision." It was a powerful way to build confidence.

Maybe you've been told all your life what to do and what's expected. Maybe that's why you've scoured the pages of this book looking for "the rules" or a convenient list of the foods you must forbid yourself. I'm not going to tell you what to eat or when to eat it. You're a big kid now (no pun intended). Instead, I'll give you some guidelines, share my own opinion, and explain possible consequences. But ultimately, it's time to rebuild your self-confidence in the diet department. You need to make some decisions yourself and gain the confidence that comes only with knowledge and experience. I think you're way too smart to have me dictate what you put in your mouth and when. I believe you will take responsibility for your eating habits and craft your own success.

The Traffic Light Approach to Food

My system of traffic light tiers allows you to quickly categorize foods as: Green means go. Red means stop. Yellow means proceed with caution. It's simple. And if you're a parent, this approach is even simple enough to share with your kids. There's no value in teaching your child that sugary juice boxes are "bad" when little Johnnie's BFF will suck down three of those bad boys during the course of a 1-hour playdate later that day. Avoid labeling food as "bad." Labeling food as a color in a three-tier system makes smart food choices far less confusing.

Each traffic light tier is a sampling of foods. Certainly from looking at the examples provided below, you can make an estimated guess as to where any food item in question might land. When in doubt, Google the food. When you're at the market, read the ingredient label or use an app to quickly assess the nutritional value of everything that lands in your cart and ultimately your body. And again . . . my system is a guideline. Feel free to decide for yourself where certain items belong. For example, when it comes to most sugar-free, calorie-free drinks, I used to think they all belonged in the Green Zone. But as I researched the effects of the food coloring and artificial sweeteners contained in these beverages, I decided to move them to my Yellow Zone.

As you will see, each zone has levels. Some types of foods are better than others, even when both types are found in the same color tier. On the lists below, the highest quality foods are listed first. There are some items on the Green Zone list that score just slightly above foods in the Yellow Zone. The higher on the Green Zone list you stay, the further away you are from the Yellow Zone.

Green Zone

Green Zone foods are the foods that provide you with optimal nutrition. These foods are the pinnacle, your ultimate goal. As a rule, you'll strive to eat from your list of Green Zone foods 80 percent or more of the time. I'm not going to dictate the foods in this zone. I can make suggestions, but remember your choices are your own: Whatever you put in this zone will be carefully selected by you!

Foods in the Green Zone should give you the nutritional power to perform at your best, look your best, and feel your best emotionally. Green Zone foods help stabilize your energy. When you look at an item of food, ask yourself this simple question: "Is this food good for me, bad for me, or meaningless to my health?" If clearly you believe the food is good for you, it goes in your personally selected Green Zone.

When you consume the healthiest of whole foods with minimal processing and proven health benefits, you dramatically improve your overall quality of life. Green Zone foods will allow you to feel greater emotional stability, have fewer cravings and fewer chronic aches and pains, and experience a whole slew of physical benefits such as better skin, shinier hair, faster-growing nails, and a better body! But perhaps most important and least discussed is the effect our nutrition has on our ability to perform mentally. The journal *Clinical Rheumatology* (July 2006) reported on a study in the United Kingdom that demonstrated that nutritional deficiencies resulted in a drastically reduced brain functioning and ability. Evidence in that study suggests that something as simple as a the right amount of vitamin D reduced levels of stress, anxiety, and depression.

Keep in mind that how you prepare your food affects which zone you place them in. Don't try to trick yourself into believing that broccoli still belongs in the Green Zone if you've coated it in thick, goopy cheese sauce. To really deserve a spot on your Green team, foods should be eaten raw, steamed, grilled, poached, baked, or broiled. Again, where you place foods is up to you, but *hel-lo,* if it's coated in butter, salt, or cream sauce or deep-fried, it really doesn't make sense to be in your Green or Yellow Zone.

Your nutritional objective should be constantly being on the hunt for foods that you love and that meet your own Green Zone standards. Remember, these are the foods you have chosen to help you live the life you deserve! Work to get 80 percent of your calories or more from your Green Zone.

MY GREEN ZONE

Water

Dark leafy greens

Dark red fruits

Dark green and vibrantly colored vegetables

Cauliflower

Dark-colored berries

Vibrantly colored thick-skinned fruits (skin on)

Chickpeas

Citrus fruits

Egg whites

Green tea

Vinegar

PB2 powdered peanut butter

Meaty fish

Fatty fish

Lean white meat (chicken and pork, with fat and skin trimmed)

Raw nuts

Black beans

Hemp seed

Flaxseed

Quinoa

Extra-virgin olive oil

Whole grains

Brown rice

Steel-cut oatmeal

Salsa

Lentils

Bran

Herbs

Scallops

Seaweed

Shrimp

Fruit without the skin

Avocado

Natural organic low-fat peanut butter

Eggplant

Olives

Low-fat feta cheese

Sprouted grain bread

Mustard

Low-sodium broth soups

Whole grain, low-sugar cereal

Dark chocolate

Hummus

Tofu

Sweet potato

Low-fat turkey chili

Buckwheat pancakes

Vegetable juice, no sugar added

Fresh squeezed juice (pulp included, no sugar added)

Black coffee

Veggie burger

Corn

Buffalo (extralean)

Truvía/Stevia sweetener

Couscous

Low-fat/sugar-free frozen yogurt

Pineapple

Mango

Carb-control instant oatmeal

Air-popped popcorn

Low-fat yogurt

Raw sugar

Yellow Zone

The Yellow Zone is where you'll place foods that range from moderately nutritious to "indifferent." In other words, this zone is for foods that might be healthy, but they have a healthier alternative that you've placed in the Green Zone. The Yellow Zone also includes foods that aren't going to hurt you in small doses but that have very little nutritional value. Let me give you a personal example. I have placed fat-free, sugar-free Jell-O at the bottom of my Yellow Zone. Yes, it has practically zero calories and zero fat, but it also has zero nutritional benefit, except that it cures my after-dinner sweet tooth. Because it does contain food colorings and ingredients not found in nature appear on the ingredient list, it's not a daily staple, and that's why I believe it belongs at the bottom of my Yellow list. However, based on your own experience and research, you may believe that even the smallest amount of red dye or artificial sweeteners are unacceptable. You might place gelatin desserts in your Red Zone. Your diet, your choice.

Keep in mind that all zones have a ranking within them. It's to be expected that down the road you may find that some of the foods you currently see as "harmless" will be better placed on your Red Zone list. As your own experience and knowledge expands, you'll be able to adjust and modify your list to suit your long-term health objectives.

MY YELLOW ZONE

Soy
Lean red meat
Low-fat dairy products
Shellfish
Almond milk
Rice milk
Refried beans (fat-free)
Lean deli meat without preservatives

Baked fries
Sushi with rice (noncrunchy)
Low-fat granola
Honey
Flavored oatmeal
Rice cakes
Low-fat dressing
Unsalted butter
Whole grain crackers
Lean lamb
Tuna salad
Whole grain pasta
Whole wheat tortillas
Low-fat baked chips
Low-fat ice cream/yogurt
Jerky
Pretzels
Low-sugar/low-fat sauces and marinades
Wine

Sugar-free/fat-free processed foods
Jams and jellies
Juice
Soft cheeses
Low-calorie beer
Ketchup
Syrup
Low-fat Cool Whip
Low-fat muffins
Nut butters
Lean bacon
Turkey bacon
Veggie dogs
Thin-crust veggie pizza
Diet soda
Zero-calorie waters/drinks with food coloring or additives
Sugar-free/fat-free gelatin desserts (like Jell-O)

Red Zone

A red light traditionally means stop, but I don't want you to think it means "never" or "don't eat this." A red light in this context is meant to make you just stop. Think of how you would approach a stop sign or a red light when a marked police car is in plain view. Instantly, you snap into a present state of mind. You take inventory of the consequences of a rolling stop. You bring all four wheels to a halt, look both ways, and proceed with caution. Think of red light food as food that requires you to come to a complete stop and evaluate the consequences.

You should eat foods in this tier very rarely. How rarely depends on your priorities and your interest in being the best possible you. The portion size and frequency of eating from this tier is a reflection of the life you want to live, how you feel about your priorities, and how much you care about the important people in your life.

You don't have to completely eliminate Red Zone foods, but if you really stop to think about it, you may find that the enjoyment of eating them is not worth the negative consequences. Cupcakes from Wonderland Bakery are a Johnson family birthday tradition. No other cupcake on the planet can measure up to a Wonderland cupcake. If I'm craving a cupcake, I'll have one, but the moment of joy I get from a cupcake that's from any bakery other than Wonderland just isn't worth it. I can't remember the last time I've had most of the Red Zone items on this list; however, there are few items that I really love from time to time. Once a year, I enjoy a slice of my Aunt Nellie's apple pie. I'd say once a month I savor a skinny margarita on date night with Bret. Most the foods in my Red Zone contain ingredients that are so foreign to my body that the thought of eating them turns my stomach. When it comes to the occasional indulgence, let's just say I'm extremely choosy. It needs to be worth the consequences! A cupcake from the corner supermarket, with its tasteless greasy icing, in my food world is not worth the calories or the gurgling belly—but I can make that choice.

No one wants to be told what to do or what to eat. But you will happily eliminate Red Zone food from your diet when you realize how gross those foods make you feel. The healthier you eat,

the less tolerance your body will have for foods in this tier. Make it your decision. Do it for you.

MY RED ZONE

Alcohol	Fast-food burgers
Chips	Fried foods
Onion rings	Ice cream
Pastries	Blended coffee drinks
Nachos	Frozen hash browns (like Tater Tots)
Breakfast sand-wiches	
Cookies	Toaster pastries (like Pop-Tarts)
Buttered popcorn	Margarine
Salty processed crackers	Cinnamon buns
Candy	Sausage
Garlic toast	Potato skins
White bread	High-sugar cereal
Salad dressings	Baked beans
Taco shells	Breaded food
Pies	Fried food
Cream-based sauces	Cake
Cream-based soups	Processed meats
Soft drinks	Creamed veggies
High fructose corn syrup	Donuts
	Pizza
Grilled cheese sandwiches	Gravy
	Hot dogs

With the tiered approach to food, you use guidelines and self-education to shape your decisions. The tiers are loosely defined here so that you can organize them *personally*.

For example, you'll see that I've placed dairy products in the Yellow Zone, because I want to proceed with caution. However, your lactose intolerance or an allergy may necessitate moving dairy to the Red Zone. As you experiment, begin to pay closer attention to the machine you're driving; as you learn and experience the consequences and rewards of your food decisions, you'll naturally move more and more food from one zone to another. For instance, lean red meat might currently exist in your tier one, the Green Zone. But as you educate yourself and learn more about your food and your body, you may decide to move lean red meat to your Yellow Zone.

Ultimately, the tiers that you assign food to is up to you. You're very intelligent. I trust you'll make the best decisions. I have many friends in fitness who categorize fat-free, sugar-free Jell-O as just as poor a choice as fried chicken with gravy. I don't agree, but that's my personal choice. Each year I learn more and more about food, and I find myself moving more "fake" foods into my personal Red Zone tier.

Just as each year new research studies expose foods previously assumed to be "safe" as actually being unhealthy choices, so too will you make your own discoveries and change your mind about the placement of certain foods in one tier or another.

If I can leave you with two timeless principles of nutrition, they are:

- The closer a food is to the state in which God produced it, the healthier it probably is.

- Everything you put in your body is a choice. All choices have consequences.

Rules of the Road

Now that you understand the traffic light approach to eating, the simple guidelines that follow can keep you safe from trouble when you're cruising along.

FOR MUCHO MOJO, CHOOSE "SMART CARBS"

To live the life you want, you need *mojo*, the energy and mental fortitude it takes to make that life happen. I define mojo as a certain type of energy that makes you feel like you can do anything. You feel confident, alive, energetic, and strong. Your nutrition will deliver energy to support your mojo!

In general, choose complex carbohydrates over simple carbs. Simple carbohydrates tend to be sugars, the type of processed or refined food that breaks down easily in the body. And the reason you want to avoid simple carbohydrates and processed sugars is because you get a quick peak or a sudden jolt of energy and then a crash, leaving you lower than where you started. You want a well-balanced level of energy that you can sustain day in and day out for the rest of your life. So avoid simple carbs. They're addictive empty calories. White-flour breads, pastas, sugars, pastries, chips, processed crunchy stuff, white rice, and most all processed foods make us crave more processed foods.

You do need carbohydrates, so chose whole grains, fruits with the skin on, and other nutrient-dense choices. Look for high-quality sources of natural complex carbohydrates, like yams or sweet potatoes—sweet potatoes could be cooked in minutes in your microwave. Be creative.

BREAK THE BREAKFAST FAST

Not sure who started this trend, but millions of Americans have adopted the habit of skipping breakfast. Not you! You're serious now, and you understand that your nutritional day will begin with a healthy breakfast. Breakfast is the best time to consume complex carbohydrates. Breakfast sets the tone for your energy and your metabolism for the entire day. When you skip breakfast and just down a cup of coffee, all you're doing is slowing your metabolism. A slower metabolism makes you feel tired and sluggish. A good breakfast can include a great source of complex carbohydrates like steel-cut oatmeal or egg whites and sprouted grain toast, or maybe a red apple with some cottage cheese and crushed almonds on top. Starting your day

From "Deprivation" to Healthy Decisions

I won't suggest you deprive yourself or eliminate certain foods, but you may decide to do that on your own, based on realizing the consequences of eating those foods. Again, I'll share my opinion, and you'll make the decision that's right for you.

As you begin to consume more and more health-supporting, highly nutritious foods, your taste for crap practically disappears. As your tastes and cravings change, you'll naturally begin to eat more nutrient-dense foods. And guess what? You will be rewarded! You'll lose weight, look great, have energy, and you'll want to learn more! That in turn motivates you to share what you're learning with others, which in turn keeps you accountable. You'll begin to pay closer attention to labels and to shop for fresh ingredients, and gradually you'll want to eliminate as much "junk fuel" as possible.

A shift will occur, a shift so slight that I must actually point it out lest you miss it or trivialize it. That shift is *autonomous choice*.

There's a difference between "depriving yourself" of a certain food and not wanting to put it in your body in the first place. Deprivation and restrictions occur when a diet dictates *for* you what you can and cannot eat. Deprivation and restrictions occur when you stop eating a food but you still want it. People trying to find control in an out-of-control life, or who punish themselves by restricting calories, often use deprivation as a form of coping with stress or as an expression of self-hate.

The switch happens when you *consciously and independently* make the decision that one food makes you look and feel better than another. That's when you stop *wanting* junk. One food helps you to live the life you want; another undermines the quality of your life. It becomes as simple as that.

with a healthy breakfast will kick your metabolism into gear. It's one of the best ways to get your mojo pumping.

EAT EVERY FEW HOURS

Now, I recommend that most people try to eat every 2½ to 3½ hours. Keep in mind, however, that everyone is different. Keep a journal next to (or on!) your phone or on your computer desktop and record when you eat, what you eat, and how your energy level feels in the following time increments: at 9:00 a.m., noon, 6:00 p.m., and 9:00 p.m. Do a little bit of personal research and experiment. Do some detective work and figure out what works best for you. But the key is maintaining a balance of small meals so that your body's never working in overdrive and expend-

Daily**PUSH**

1. Create your own Green, Yellow, and Red Zone lists. Feel free to use my categories as your guide, but begin by listing all of your favorite foods and the foods that have become staples of your diet and place them honestly in the zone in which you believe they belong. There are plenty of resources online that can give you the scoop on whether something is truly healthful or whether it's packed with hidden sugars and calories. The ingredient label is always a good place to start.

2. For the next several days, each time you have a meal, snack, or beverage, pull out your lists and make a note of which zone you're eating or drinking from.

NOTES

_____

_____

_____

_____

_____

_____

ing too much energy breaking down your food.

By dividing your day into small manageable meals—that's five, six, maybe even seven meals a day—I think you're going to find a much more balanced level of energy throughout the day. The honest truth is, I sometimes I get so caught up in whatever I'm doing that I need to place a reminder alarm on my phone to eat every 3 hours.

MAKE SIMPLE CUTS

One of the easiest ways to cut 200 or 300 calories a day from your diet is to cut something you always have but wouldn't really miss. Chose a food or drink that has simply become a habit—

not something you crave, but something rather irrelevant. That way, when you cut it, you won't feel deprived. A sugary blended coffee drink might taste nice on my drive to the office, but can I do without it? Definitely. Simple solution. If you happen to adore your sugary blended coffee drink and cannot imagine how you'd get through your morning without it, might I suggest trying one of the lower-calorie "skinny" alternatives?

Or how about choosing between mayo or cheese on your sandwich? Get rid of one, and you'll save about 100 calories. Give your own diet the once-over, and I'll bet you can find several cuts that will cause zero feelings of deprivation.

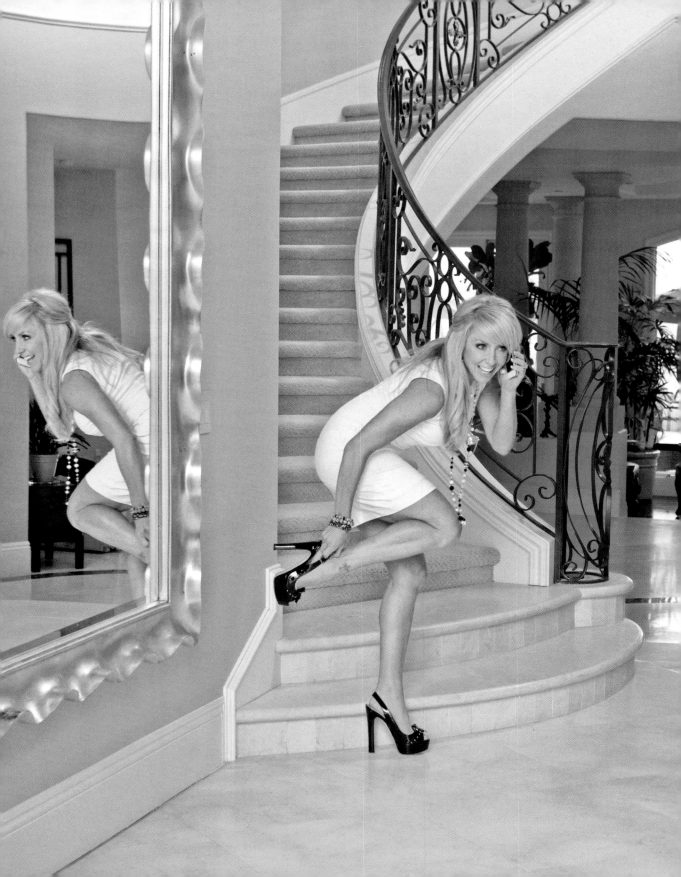

DAY 18

Add **MORE HOURS** to Your Day

A Few Simple Habits to Help You Master Your Time

The number-one excuse for skipping exercise is (drumroll, please): *"I don't have enough time!"* Well, today you learn how to find more of it!

We're all stuck with the same 24 hours in a day. So it's not time management that we need to improve, it's *personal* management. The system you'll learn today teaches you not how to do *more* but what to do *less of* so that you can make most productive use of your time.

The fact that someone as busy as you has carved out the time to read this book says that you're probably one of the most organized people you know. But if you wish to be even more productive, that requires changing or improving just a few of your habits—incremental, manageable habits that you can begin today.

If you want to move faster in your career, improve your business, have more time for your family, friends, or fitness pursuits, then you have no choice but to develop habits that allow you to make better use of your time. Today you will.

Productivity doesn't mean working more, it means being alert to opportunities to better use every moment. And time management isn't about creating more hours in the day, it's about getting in the habit of scheduling your day in a way that allows you to honor your priorities and get to the important stuff! As you'll see, exercise is the key.

Energy Equals Productivity

We can't manufacture more hours for our day, but we can be infinitely productive with the time we do have. To be more productive, you need more *umph!*

The number-one way to improve your physical energy, mental stamina, work performance, focus, and ability to cope with stress is exercise. Just exercise.

Don't take my word for it! There's a mountain of research to support my enthusiastic review. In fact, the American College of Sports Medicine found that the productivity of people after exercise was an average of 65 percent higher than those who did not exercise.

If I have something that's really bothering me, so much that it almost hurts my head to try to sort it out, I always find the solution in a puddle of sweat! Intense exercise is like taking a magic pill that gives you the ability to solve problems like a superhero. This "intense exercise" is defined individually based on your level of fitness. Intense for one person might be sprinting on a treadmill; for someone less conditioned, it might be walking at her fastest pace for 20 minutes.

But to fit in exercise, you need to get your personal time management together. Here's my three-step system that helps you do it.

Step One: Ask Yourself the Golden Question

To improve your use of time, ask yourself this simple question throughout the day: "Is this the most important thing I can be doing right now and the most valuable use of my time?"

The answer is always clear. Now I'm not going to pretend to be perfectly productive. Sure, there are times you might find me enjoying a little train-wreck TV, gluing rhinestones to an inanimate object, or even admiring the vacation photos of someone I don't know on Facebook. An outsider might smirk and say, "Is that *really* the best use of your time?"

YES! Sometimes the best of use of time is to let your brain chill. Vacations, hobbies, lying on

You Snooze, You Lose

When you set your alarm, don't hit Snooze. Instead, put your alarm so far from your bed that you are forced to actually get up and turn it off. As soon as goes off, begin repeating to yourself, "I'm up! I'm up! I'm up!"

It works!

the floor with your 5-year-old, and even the occasional nap are all important and necessary to have a well-balanced life. Your exceptional planning will allow this freedom.

Step Two: Reverse Engineer Your Day

According to time management experts, people who spend 10 minutes a day planning save themselves 1½ to 3 hours for each of those 10-minute blocks of time. Leaving your day and the hours you have available to chance guarantees you will lose track of your time and sabotage your own productivity.

Your time is much more valuable than the money you have in your bank. So you want to spend it, use it, allocate it wisely.

SET YOUR PRIORITIES The most basic step in planning your day is to set your priorities. Your priorities determine what must be done today and which activities have the greatest impact on your health and Push goals.

The first items on your Today list are those which *must* be done today to avoid negative consequences. (In other words, if they don't get done today, there will be hell to pay.) Those are the items that go on my Today list—and exercise always makes the cut.

After priorities come additional items that move you closer to achieving your health and Push goals.

Don't add the list of tasks you "hope" to get to. If you utilize this system, you will eventually get to these "hope tos"—but you must stick to this system. If you try to cheat it, those items will continue to stockpile.

CREATE BLOCKS OF TIME FOR EACH ACTION ITEM Look at the items on your to-do list that *must* be done today, including exercise, food prep, and actions that move you closer to your Push goal. Assign a block of time to them. Be realistic about how long items will take. Make room for the unexpected, and cushion your estimate generously. Padding your estimates will allow you to deal with life's unexpected chaos.

SCHEDULE EACH BLOCK ON YOUR CALENDAR Next, pull out your calendar. This step is where you actually schedule your day. *("I pray you're keeping that on your phone," she said, palms together, eyes looking toward the heavens.)*

Now listen, I'm fine if you sketch this out on paper first, but ultimately it needs to be on your phone. Your schedule has to be with you at all times, so let's get in the habit sooner rather than later and start using the calendar on our phones.

Step Three: Get Moving Early

When I tell people that I work out at 5:30 a.m., they invariably look at me like I have lost my marbles. They always say, "I couldn't do that. I'm not a morning person." And I always say, "Neither am I!" But I have studied the habits of the successful. One common attribute of successful people is that they tend to exercise before they start their workday.

Successful people begin their day earlier than the rest. They recognize that exercise enhances their productivity and energy level.

One of the reasons you've made it to Day 18 is that you want to live a fuller life and spend more time with the people you love. If you're scheduling your health and fitness at 5:00 or 6:00 p.m. or after work, for starters you may be

Find Creative Ways to Get Moving

Let me share with you my favorite way to multitask. Several years ago, I invested in a used recumbent bike. You can find a great recumbent bike with very little wear on it. (We've all probably bought fitness equipment, only to let it gather dust in the garage.) While most days I'm going to ask you to exercise at a pace that is considered intense, a good number of days your objective will simply be to get your heart pounding for a solid 30 minutes or more.

I call this workout the executive workout. I've convinced many an entrepreneur to exercise by giving them permission to indulge in their inbox addiction. While peddling on a recumbent bike, you can very easily return e-mails, text messages, or create your to-do list. Productivity at its finest!

As a matter of fact, I'm happy to admit that fully 50 percent of this book was written while I was pedaling on my recumbent bike! Who wants to be a slug in a chair for thousands of hours?

I found a fabulous little contraption called a "lap desk" from Amazon.com that allows me to position my laptop in an ergonomic position for typing while I ride. There have been days that I just pedaled through 3 hours of writing. I don't pedal at a breakneck pace, just enough to keep me alert with my heart rate raised slightly so I can be fully engaged in my writing. By my Fitbit calculations, I burn nearly twice the number of calories while pedaling slowly than I do while writing in my office chair. I've also found that my creativity and passion for my writing increased while I was actively using my muscles.

Give it a whirl! Every gym has recumbent bikes! I'm sure you're clever enough to rig up a laptop setup that works for you. Or simply work with a smaller portable device, like your phone, iPad, or tablet.

spending even more time away from your loved ones. And both of us know that inevitably something always comes up after 5:00 p.m. that makes it nearly impossible for you to stick to your exercise routine.

I want to push you to develop the habit of exercising before you begin your day. For some, that's 5:00 a.m.; for others, it might be 8:00 a.m. Whether you're a stay-at-home mom or a dude in a suit, there's an hour at which your day's official business begins.

I know it's early. I ain't gonna lie; it's hell for about 6 seconds when that alarm blares at 4:45 a.m.! But as soon as my feet hit the ground, it's all good! When you exercise at that hour, the people who you care about are still sleeping, so you're not missing anything.

I encourage you to give it a try for one week.

Daily**PUSH**

1. Get in the habit of asking yourself, "Is this the most effective use of my time right now?"

2. List your activities for tomorrow.

3. Estimate the time each will take.

4. Use your calendar to block the time for each.

5. Set your alarm for tomorrow's preworkday workout!

NOTES

_____

_____

_____

_____

_____

_____

You will find you'll have more energy, experience greater productivity and improved clarity, and actually feel good about yourself! You'll be able to eradicate the looming pressure of an impending workout at the end of the day when you are truly exhausted.

You Are *Not* Too Tired (Trust Me)!

Aside from not having enough time, the second most popular excuse for skipping workouts is having low energy.

I have a great energy-boosting resource for you! (Insert evil laugh . . . *Muuhhaaa-ha-ha!*) Exercise *gives* you energy! And it's not just my pushy opinion or even my experience with thousands of people that proves this to be true. There are actual white-lab-coat-wearing smart people who have research that confirms it!

In addition to everything else, early-morning exercise will give you higher energy at midday. This extra midday energy helps to curb your appetite and promotes the mental acuity you need to get yourself off of Facebook and on to something that moves you closer to your Push goal!

People, we have a life to create here!

By adapting the habit of an early-morning exercise routine, you might experience the following side effects: improved fitness, younger appearance, increased self-confidence, heightened sex drive, longer life span, improved quality of life, weight loss, and greater time productivity.

All that and you're telling me you're going to "try" to wake up an hour earlier to do this? "I'll try" is not going to fly with me. Come on! You and I both know that "I'll try" translates to "I will set my alarm to go off early, but I've already made up my mind that I will hit Snooze and go back to sleep."

Don't you dare tell me you're going to try. You have to *promise* you will do this! Better yet, take action right this second. Grab your phone and text a friend who will meet you for your workout. Text your partner, your best friend, a personal trainer, the gym manager . . . I don't care who you text, but tell someone right now that he or she can expect to see you bright and early tomorrow morning!

I told you I was pushy!

But I would never push you to do something I didn't believe in 100 percent. You have nothing to lose, except maybe a few pounds.

DAY 19

On a Diet versus
HAVING A DIET

There's a Huge Difference!

You've already redefined success. Today we'll redefine diet. But first let me tell you a story.

Shortly after I signed my first infomercial deal, I found myself in the office of one of the company's nutritional experts. His task was to take notes and research the diet I had used to help thousands of people lose weight under my kickboxing program, Turbo Kick. In my lap was my "big book"— a ginormous folder I had assembled over the past 4 or 5 years of before-and-after photos. The book became notorious in the infomercial world, as it was filled with pages of people who had sent their pictures to me documenting their weight loss of 50, 60, 90, 100, and even 200 pounds. Picture after picture of regular folks who, frankly, looked nothing like the people in their before photos.

Steve had pulled out a pad of paper to take notes on our conversation. "So, tell me about the parameters of the diet you had them follow," he said with a smile, pencil pressed to the pad, ready to scribble away.

"I didn't give them a diet," I answered sheepishly. I wondered if my honesty might cost me the deal. "I just suggested that people adopt a diet, a way of eating they could sustain. You know, treat yourself like a lifelong athlete."

"Great!" he replied. "But the bottom line is the people who pick up the phone when they see your spot on TV want rules, lots of structure, and your special formula. People want you to tell them what to eat, when to eat, and why to eat it. And . . . they'll need a time frame. They'll need to know how long they have to do this for."

What he was sharing with me was the truth about marketing. Diets sell. Most people want you to do the work for them. They want rules.

137

They want restrictions and limits, definitions and portions. Those who are trapped in the mind-set of dieting need structure and a finish line.

Do you see why I told you that story? I think you're too smart to fall for that over and over again!

In my obsession to reveal the difference between lifelong dieters and those who seem to effortlessly maintain a healthy weight and fitness levels, I've noticed something: The key distinction between these two types of people is their understanding of the word *diet*—and the way they use the "d-word" results from the habits they've formed around food.

Today, you decide which type of person you want to be: a chronic dieter or a person who can manage a healthy weight and live harmoniously with food. (Hint: It's the second one!)

Restrictive Diets *Do* Work (Sort Of)

We're forever hearing in books or in the media that "diets don't work." But as a fitness professional, I know saying that damages my credibility, because diets *do* work—if your goal is to *temporarily* lose weight.

In fact, the phase "diets don't work" might be doing more harm than good; anyone who has ever gone on a diet before knows that if she follows the diet, it works!

Dieting doesn't work *long term* might be a more accurate phrase. Restricting calories for prolonged periods will help you lose weight, but here's another truth: Eventually, you'll gain all of it back and then some.

In short, any temporary diet (or "dieting" versus having a healthy lifestyle) sets you up for failure. Ever heard of the dangers of losing precious muscle mass when on these diets, instead of losing the fat? How about losing muscle from the heart? Slowing your metabolism? Stripping the joy from food? No thanks. Restrictive diets can be damaging to your metabolism, muscle maintenance, and worst of all, your confidence.

Being a "Dieter" Fuels Deprivation, Desperation, and Doubt

The dieter establishes strict rules, beliefs, and self-imposed deprivation. Deprivation creates intense desire and forces a battle of will. As the desire builds and resolve fades, you feel failure is near. In walks a bad day and a glass of wine. Now inhibitions are low and reckless abandonment is only a pantry away. As the forbidden food makes its way into the dieter's no-try zone, it's on like Donkey Kong! A loaf of bread and a chocolate cake later, the dieter is now either off the diet or determined to punish herself by eating nothing but an apple for the next 3 days.

Dieters go through life labeling food as either "good" or "bad" and can't find a balance. They think the term *moderation* is only for genetic carriers of the "skinny" chromosome; it doesn't apply to those who diet. Food is a constant preoccupation and a never-ending battle that causes hormonal imbalance, stress, and an obsession with weight. Diet is king, the scale rules the empire, and food is the enemy.

Dieters are always second-guessing themselves, wondering if they ate too much or the right foods. Dieters plan their day around what they cannot eat.

"Having a Diet" Fuels Careful Eating

My friend Toni Cook, superfit mother of seven, is a great example of a person who *has* a diet. I became friends with Toni in 2005 when she started taking my Turbo Kick classes to get back in shape after the quads (yes, *quads!*) had started preschool. It wasn't long before we became friends and I asked her to be in several of my fitness videos. If you own any of my workouts, you can probably spot her in many of them. Toni is one of those people who are often accused by "dieters" of being able to eat whatever they want.

Maybe it was her tradition of celebrating the end of each video production with an order of Carl's Jr. chili-cheese fries. The cameramen, craft service people, and crew would all sneer knowingly, "Oh, that it explains it! She can eat anything she wants!" or "Wow! If I ate like that, I would weigh 300 pounds."

But the truth is that Toni, and the rest of the video talent, had just finished *8 hours* of intense cardiovascular effort in take after take for the video. For the day in total, I suspect she burned about 4,500 calories—or more. Chili-cheese fries come in around 800 calories and with 40 grams of fat. Ouch! But in the grand scheme of things, she had room in her calorie allotment for the day to eat 5 or 6 large orders. *(Gagging at the thought of it . . .)*

Though genetically freakish people do exist

(and we have an obligation to at least be nice to them), as a rule of thumb, when you see a healthy, fit individual enjoying a food that you have labeled as bad, the truth is likely that they are savoring a rare splurge.

Careful eaters know when they've had enough and when they can afford to have a little extra. To the outsider, it might look like they can eat whatever they want, but the reality is that someone who *has* a diet is a habitually healthy or clean eater. It's a habit, not an obsession.

Recently, while at a large dinner party, I was seated next to a young woman I had met for the first time that evening. When the servers offered our final course for the night, German chocolate cake, I politely declined. By this point, I had already noticed she was studying every bite I put in my mouth. "Ohhhhh, you don't eat cake, right?" she asked, as if to validate the assumptions she had formed. "No, I eat cake," I replied, "if I'm craving it."

I knew my answer didn't quite add up for her. It wasn't the time of the place to go into a detailed explanation. Dieters want rules. Hard-and-fast rules to live by.

"Having a Diet" Allows Food to Be a Pleasure

Dieters' food choices are in constant flux. For them, one month carbs are the enemy, and the next month they're surviving on fruit smoothies or their own version of a liquid diet.

When the chronic dieter is not in "diet" mode, however, all bets are off. Even the foods that they themselves have labeled bad become fair play. But when the dieter is on active diet duty, they dare not take even a bite. Just 1 teaspoon of ice cream might cause them to slide down a slippery slope.

Someone who *has a diet* can delight in a shared brownie sundae with a group of friends. The brownie doesn't control the spoon, and food doesn't limit their joy.

When dieters actually diet, pleasure and food do not coexist. Their only objective when preparing and eating food is to ensure that meals comply with their diet rules. Careful eaters habitually enjoy foods that serve their nutritional and physical requirements as part of their regular diet. They look forward to their meals, and though some foods are a considered a rare treat, nothing is all-out banned. A few bites can satisfy, nullifying the temptation to overindulge.

A careful eater's experience with food is based on the knowledge that he or she has control. These eaters know their numbers (approximately) and they keep a general idea of where they're at. They know how certain foods make them feel, and they eat to perform their best. Quite simply, careful eaters are confident in the way they eat.

How to Transition from Dieting to Having a Diet

Yes, we are talking about changing your thinking. And as I've said many times in this book, I personally have found that it is easier for people to first change their habits, and then the new thinking follows as a natural progression. You can change the way you think about the word *diet*. It's a process. It's a series of habits. Tomorrow we'll go into great detail about those habits. But today you begin by uncovering and reprocessing your relationship to the word and the definition you've given it.

The first step in the transition: deciding to make the transition! This process starts with a decision to use a different definition. You've got 10 seconds to decide . . . what will you chose? Are you *on* a diet or will you commit to *having* a diet, a diet that you enjoy and can realistically maintain the rest of your life?

Good choice! Now you're ready to have a diet. Here the steps you'll take.

LEARN ABOUT NUTRITION Educate yourself on the nutritional value of food. Learn how each food will benefit your body. An open-minded approach to learning can accelerate your transition. As you learn about food, the body, and how negatively our dieting approaches have affected our bodies, you will begin to put new habits into practice. These new habits will give you instant gratification. Your positive success will motivate you to learn even more.

CONTINUE TO EXPLORE YOUR GOALS AND PRIORITIES To change the way you feel about food, you need to change the way you feel about yourself. To change the way you feel about yourself, you need to know who you are, what you want, and how you will get it; then you have to do something about it! Reading this book is a great start.

Your relationship with food is a reflection of your sense of self-worth. It will improve as you align your eating and physical activity with your goals and priorities. Success is defined in terms of how these changes make you feel about yourself.

CONFRONT YOUR CORE ISSUES Randomly eating and severely restricting food to manage your emotions and distract yourself from unpleasant thoughts—this is what really needs to be addressed. You have to learn to take good care of yourself by creating a successful foundation. Addressing emotional needs, past traumas, and years of restricting or overeating requires a commitment to seeking professional help and a commitment to learn to love yourself. (Remember, you cannot give what you do not have. You have people who deserve your love, but you must have it for yourself first.)

Change is possible. It starts with your decision to learn more and change your habits.

Daily PUSH

1. Review the list of goals you've made for yourself this year.

2. Each time you have a negative thought about a food or food choice, remind yourself that you *have* a healthy diet, but you're not *on* a diet.

3. Educate yourself. Spend 20 minutes today researching more about the healthiest foods available to you and about a lifestyle diet that you can subscribe to for the rest of your life.

NOTES

_____

_____

_____

_____

_____

_____

FOCUS ON ACTIONS, NOT EMOTIONS A positive change in your thinking will happen as you begin to change your behavior. I know you've heard the opposite, but my experience in helping thousands of people adopt this way of thinking has taught me that change comes easiest when you start with the behavior. Changing our minds is our ultimate goal, but with discipline we can change our behaviors tomorrow. When your behaviors change, your results will improve. Your positive results will naturally change your thinking.

Ultimately, Happiness Is What We Crave

It's only human to want to be your best or to maintain a healthy weight. Show me someone who doesn't think that he or she could stand to lose a few pounds. But when a preoccupation with weight or appearance takes over your thoughts, consumes your behavior, zaps the joy out of eating, and damages your relationships, *you've gotta wake up*. Aside from the health consequences of what you're doing, consider the effect on your happiness. Reaching the "perfect" number on a scale will not bring you happiness.

Take a look again at the 10 goals you set for yourself this year. The ones that result in more time and closeness with the people you love are the goals that will ultimately bring you happiness. You selected each one of your goals because, when accomplished, you believe this goal will make you happy. Reaching and maintaining a healthy weight, free of the dieter's mentality, will bring you peace. Reaching the perfect weight through a series of calorie-restrictive, food-banning, joy-depriving, unrealistic diets might make your jeans a little looser, but it will not bring you joy.

There is more than one way to get to the where you want to be. The way that will bring you the most peace and joy is learning *to have* a diet.

10 **EATING HABITS** of the Highly Successful and Fit

The Secrets That Take You from Fat to Fit

Successfully fit people are successful not because of good luck, birth order, or family heritage but because they have adopted the right habits. They do things differently than the rest. While some of them keep their habits covered up like the answers to a test, I've spoken to thousands of successful people who feel obliged to share their practices with others. So today, I share with you what they have shared with me.

To be a successful person, you must adopt the habits of success.

Stephen Covey's theories on learning from the habits of successful people in his book *The*

Seven Habits of Highly Effective People suggest that by emulating the habits of successful people, anyone can enjoy the life he or she desires. Learn the habits, adopt the habits, practice the habits, enjoy the success. It really is that basic.

You're not going to find the stuff in this chapter that you might find on the cover of a magazine. There's a slew of information in health magazines written by dietitians and nutritionists about what we are supposed to do that has nothing in common with what naturally healthy eaters really do. I wanted to uncover the habits of those who do it effortlessly—regardless of whether it was sexy, interesting, or even appropriate.

On the menu today: an unbiased look into the eating habits of highly successful fit people. Here I've done the hard part: I've compiled secrets from thousands of successfully fit. I had to. Children learn from their parents and the environment in which they were raised. And um, well, if you actually read my intro, you know that gas station cuisine was a staple in my household when I was growing up. I had to study fit people. I needed to learn these habits. Now I share them with you!

1. They Tend to Stick to the Same "Daily Menu"

I'll go out on a limb and tell you something that approximately zero weight-loss experts are willing to share with you. If you Google "weight loss tips" or "healthy eating habits," nearly every blog and article you find will suggest that you "eat a variety of healthy foods to prevent boredom." Undoubtedly, eating a variety of foods may very

well be exciting. But my job is to tell you what fit people do, not what they should do or what sounds good to a registered dietitian.

Astrid Boetel is one of many people I've interviewed on the subject. At 60-plus years young, she still wears micro shorts and midriff-baring bra tops that reveal her amazingly defined abs. Astrid explained to me, "I basically eat the same thing for most meals. When I go out to dinner or eat with friends, I also try to eat healthy, but I love trying new foods."

I've spent nearly 20 years studying people with exceptional eating habits, and this particular habit was perhaps one of the most telling. The majority tell me they eat virtually the same meals every day, mostly the same breakfast, same lunch, same dinner, and when it comes to snacks and beverages . . . well, you guessed it, very predictable food. To clarify, they did not suggest that they eat exactly the same entree for every meal, but they often chose from three, maybe four things that they like for breakfast, lunch, and dinner. For months on end, mealtime feels something a bit like the film *Groundhog Day*.

Whether I was speaking to fellow fitness professionals, those who have been trim all their lives, or individuals who had succeeded at taking off 100-plus pounds and keeping it off for years, this one habit always came to bear. For me, it was reassuring. I'm a creature of habit. I too like to have the very same thing for breakfast day after day after day. As I drive home from the gym at 6:30 a.m., I'm delighted to enjoy my first meal of the day. It's not a chore or a "Oh, I have to eat *that* again." Rather, it's something I quite look forward to.

I have my own theories about this shared habit. First, it allows "careful" eaters to predict their daily calorie allotment without much effort. Second, perhaps the most fit among us are entrenched in habit, including the habit of taste. Third, effortlessly fit folks are in tune with the energy and calorie needs of their bodies. When they find foods that deliver what they need and that they enjoy, why look further? Keep in mind, there's a fine line between careful eating and disordered eating. The careful eater's diet is a habit and not a matter of control or obsession.

2. They Eat Breakfast

This one common characteristic is not only universal in my experience, it's nearly universal in statistical studies of people who have achieved and maintained a large weight loss. Eighty percent of those who have been able to maintain a weight loss of at least 30 pounds for at least a year report that they always eat breakfast. Research has consistently shown that the people who successfully lose weight are the ones that wake up and eat! Furthermore, people who eat breakfast regularly have better vitamin and mineral status and eat fewer calories from fat. Experts agree that the majority of people who struggle with overeating are those who *undereat* during the first part of the day, specifically those who skip breakfast. So it seems that breakfast really is the most important meal of the day!

Why does eating breakfast help people lose and ultimately maintain a healthier weight? One theory suggests that eating a healthy breakfast reduces hunger throughout the rest of the day, therefore decreasing the likelihood of overeating and making poor food choices at lunch.

3. They Drink Water

Not soda. Not iced tea. Just plain old water. This is the biggie. Drinking enough water is a vital part of any conditioning program because it keeps your body functioning in homeostasis and aids every aspect of bodily function. Highly successful fit people drink *at least* six to eight 12-ounce glasses of water a day, plus more as needed during exercise. *Note:* It's possible to drink *too* much water, which dilutes the body's electrolytes (potassium, sodium, chloride, magnesium). Don't drink more than a gallon a day unless you're also replenishing your electrolytes.

4. They Eat Small—And Often

Most people know that small, frequent meals are absolutely the only way to go. Why? Because when we go longer than 3 hours without eating, our levels of the stress hormone cortisol rise. And high cortisol levels signal the body to store fat in the abdominal region. Keep in mind too that people who skip meals have the highest cortisol levels of all!

Eating small meals more often reduces cortisol levels, research suggests. In a study published in the *New England Journal of Medicine*, people who ate six small meals a day for 2 weeks, as opposed to three large meals containing the same total number of calories, reduced their cortisol levels by more than 17 percent! They lost belly fat, too.

When you eat small, frequent meals long term, the body becomes efficient at keeping cortisol levels low, which helps both men and women reduce belly fat.

Eating throughout the day also makes you less tempted by the monster-size buckets of popcorn and supersize fries and drink containers that include triple and quadruple servings. Guided by their nutritional needs and deeply rooted habit to eat small meals throughout the day, the superfit stand steadfast, even in the face of a delicious, jumbo chocolate-chip muffin.

5. They Eat Whole Foods First

Successful fit people tend to eat mainly whole, unprocessed foods, including fruits, veggies, and whole grains (and products made from whole grains). Certainly they enjoy the occasional treat, but 80 percent of the time or more,

Tipping Equals Good Karma

Good manners go a long way, but a nice tip is always appreciated. Having been a waitress for many years (including a stint in a brown polyester shift dress at Bob's Big Boy), I can confirm that it behooves you to get your server on your side right off the bat! Give 'em a heads-up: "I promise I'm a great tipper, but I'm hoping you can help me with a special order."

Don't be afraid to ask that things be prepared in a way that places your nutritional needs first. There's no need to feel embarrassed by asking for something that's not on the menu. If you see that certain ingredients are in other entrees, I bet with your charm, and with your server as your liaison, you can "getter done"! What's the worst thing that could happen? Your server might say no? Nope. It could be much worse. Fail to ask, and your healthy, boneless breast of chicken may be served to you in buttery cream sauce concealing 50 grams of fat. There's nothing to be embarrassed by, unless yo mamma never taught you your manners or you're a cheapskate when it comes to tipping! Remember . . . good tip equals good karma!

their preference leads to whole foods.

Whole, natural foods—apples, steel-cut oatmeal, broccoli, salads, brown rice—are what food researchers call *low-density* foods. That is, they take up a lot of room in your stomach because they contain lots of fiber, which satisfies hunger with few calories. *High-density* foods are the opposite; they are things like butter, oils, candy, or ice cream. Think about how much frosting you could pack into your stomach if you really tried. (Okay, don't think about it—it's too gross.) Eating mostly low-density foods is the easiest way to keep your weight in check without feeling hungry or like you're depriving yourself.

6. They Know Their Foods

This characteristic is truly universal among fit people: They know, generally speaking, every food's calories and approximate protein, carbohydrate, and fat content. It's not a case of being idiot savants but rather of having an understanding, a knowledge of food that allows them to make an educated guess. Their assumptions are almost always spot-on. This gift affords them the skill of making better food choices on a moment's notice.

Just as important: They know what one serving of said food really looks like. You can show an effortlessly fit person a whole grain cracker, and even without looking at the label, he or she can accurately predict how many crackers count as one serving. It's not a gift, actually. It's a skill, and all habits are skills you can master.

This skill is easier to acquire than it sounds. A couple of weeks of label reading is all it takes. There are even apps for your phone and Web sites that provide this information quickly and for free.

Fit people are knowledge seekers. They respect the temperamental nature of this magnificent machine that we call the human body. In the same way you would select the highest grade of gas when fueling your sports car, fit folks select a certain grade of nutrition.

Now, I won't tell you that these fit-for-life types walk around reading every label or interrogating the host at a dinner party. They do, however, have an interest, a level of knowledge about food and its nutritional value. They have a curiosity, a protective approach of selecting the best fuel for their bodies.

7. They Eat Their Favorite Foods— Carefully

Despite knowing everything about their foods and tending to stick to the same foods day in and day out, fit people rarely report eliminating foods. If it's something they crave, they enjoy a little taste. They know that simply eliminating foods they absolutely love will only set them up to fail when the temptation is too great. Instead, successfully fit people know that it's okay to indulge every once in a while. They savor those moments instead of sucking down the food as if they're afraid it's the only time they'll ever see it again.

8. They Don't Keep Red Zone Food in the House

If you look in a successfully fit person's fridge, pantry, or cupboards, you won't typically find cookies, crackers, chips, chocolate, full-fat ice cream, or soda. Why? Because they don't crave these things. They also know you can't eat 'em if you don't have 'em. Smart, right?

What's interesting about these trim types is that they don't have the same inner battle of healthy versus junkie foods that the average person who struggles with weight might have. They can walk past the aisle with chips and sodas and think nothing of it. Either they

Daily PUSH

1. Choose 5 of the 10 healthy habits listed above that you can begin practicing immediately.

2. Add a note to your smartphone's reminder system for each of these habits. (If you're not using your smartphone yet to keep track of your calendar, write a reminder of these new habits on stickie notes and post them in your kitchen!)

Special note: It's important for me to mention that there's a fine line between careful eating and disordered eating. People who are conscientious about the way they eat will try new foods and will enjoy eating healthy; food doesn't control their every thought or interfere with their joy for people and good food. Someone with a disordered way of thinking must eat the same foods every day, at every meal, and when that food is not available, they won't eat. They fear food. They use food to establish control in their lives, though ironically, ultimately it's the food that has control.

If you believe you might have an eating disorder or suspect that someone you love has gone too far, the best thing you can do is to seek professional help.

NOTES

_____

_____

_____

never developed the junk food habit or they kicked it.

9. They Close the Kitchen after Dinner

Unlike most Americans, successfully fit people eat their final meal at a reasonable hour, as opposed to eating dinner followed by a lavish 10:00 p.m. snack and another dessert. Most often they go to sleep, not hungry, but on an empty stomach. This allows them to wake up feeling thin, rested, and hungry for breakfast. It may take a little effort, but going to bed earlier and going to sleep without food awaiting digestion in your stomach keeps your body's metabolism in a fat-burning state. Instead of digesting, which causes restless sleep, your body can focus on other things—like repairing cells!

10. They're Resourceful and Politely Picky at Restaurants

Successfully fit people find healthful alternatives to selections on any menu, from a five-star restaurant's to Wendy's. They know that it's the food choices, not necessarily the restaurant choices, that help them to stay slim and healthy.

They generally steer clear of fried meat, poultry, and fish. Instead, they order their protein broiled, steamed, stir-fried, or poached. They also speak up in restaurants, politely making special requests like asking that their dish be prepared with little or no butter or sauces and with dressings on the side.

The **80/20** Rule

No Perfection Necessary (Hallelujah!!)

We've all heard of the 80/20 rule as it pertains to business, sales, and productivity. But did you know that its application is universal? It is. What you might *not* know is that you'll need to *reverse it* when it comes to your health and fitness.

Today you'll learn the advantage of applying the 80/20 rule to your Push goal, and how to flip the application of the rule to apply it to your health and fitness objectives so that it puts you on the fast track to long-term success.

The Pareto Principle

The Pareto principle states that 80 percent of all effects come from 20 percent of all causes. Vilfredo Pareto, the originator of this rule, noticed it first when studying the economic divide in society: He found that roughly 20 percent of the population owned 80 percent of all land and wealth. He began applying this principle to other categories and found the 80/20 ratio in many other situations.

Think about whether this principle is true for you. With rare exceptions, you will find that 20 percent of everything you do is responsible for 80 percent of your success. So to achieve success with the least amount of wasted effort and time, you first need to identify the 20 percent that is getting results.

How the 80/20 Rule Applies to Your Push Goal

Many believe that the 80/20 rule is universal as it relates to finances, productivity, and business. Since it is likely that your Push goal relates in some way to money or financial security, here are a few examples of the 80/20 rule as it relates to your financial productivity:

- Eighty percent of your profits will come from 20 percent of your customers.

- Since wealth is distributed in the 80/20 rule, it only makes sense that sales would follow the same course. If 20 percent of the population has more money, those same financially secure customers are the ones who will become your best customers.

- Eighty percent of your work problems will come from an area that comprises only 20 percent of your total work.

- Expect that a good 80 percent of your customer complaints will come from 20 percent of your customers.

- Twenty percent of your team will account for 80 percent of your success.

- Twenty percent of the items on your to-do list will result in 80 percent of your progress.

- Eighty percent of your ideas will keep you afloat. Twenty percent of them will take you to the next level.

- Even though you're giving 100 percent of yourself, 80 percent of your income this year will come from 20 percent of your effort.

Identify the 20 Percent That *Counts*

This concept is useful as it relates to your Push and health and fitness goals. Certain actions, perhaps an amount nearing 20 percent, will bring you much closer to your Push goal than the other 80 percent. These more-efficient actions should take highest priority when you map and revise your course.

This doesn't mean you ignore the other 80 percent once you've established which actions are most effective. It *does* mean, however, that when you ask yourself "Is this the most important thing I could be doing right now?" your most impactful activities should be on your short list.

Remember: You can't do everything. Get really good at doing the important stuff first.

My friend Brian Tracy, author of more than 60 books on productivity and goal setting, says that "once my clients understand the principle of cause and effect in their businesses, success followed soon after." Why is this so? Well, if according to the 80/20 rule, only 20 percent of your efforts (and products and staff) are the most valuable assets to your business, you can make sure that you focus on the 20 percent as your highest priority.

About 2 years before writing this book, Bret and I decided to apply this law to our area promotions directors (APDs)—i.e., our trainers and presenters. These guys and gals are independent contractors who represent our exercise and training programs in their respective states. They schedule, promote, and train others how to become fitness leaders. They are also responsible for on-site sales and registrations and for developing an ongoing personal relationship with our customers. We have criteria to evalute their success based on myriad factors, including the number of events scheduled per year, participant feedback, sales, and number of registrants, to name a few. In short, the APDs are our front line.

We established a system to evaluate which of our APDs were having the greatest effect on our business. Sure enough, just as Pareto predicted,

20 percent of them were responsible for 80 percent of our success.

Lightbulb!

Now certainly the number of sales or events that one of our APDs has versus another doesn't make that person less or more important as people. It did, however, tell us which APDs we needed to watch and learn from. It told us where to focus our praise and recognition and allowed us to better study their successful habits.

80/20 and Your To-Dos and Goals

The great thing about the 80/20 rule is that it can be universally applied to any aspect of your productivity. By now, you've probably figured out that when we went through your list of 10 goals for the next 12 months, I asked you to select one or two goals that would produce the greatest momentum in making all the other goals possible. Sound familiar? Yup (*you guessed it*), it was your Push goal. You determined it by reviewing your complete list of goals, applying the 80/20 principle, and selecting the 20 percent that make the others possible.

In the same vein, when you make your daily to-do list, if you have 10 items on that list, one or two will create the greatest momentum toward your Push goal, even if every item takes the same amount of time.

You don't have to be some big shot in the business world to make the 80/20 rule work for you! But when you apply the 80/20 rule to your Push goal, the likelihood of becoming a big shot is much greater.

As you'll see, the 80/20 rule can also help you succeed at your health and fitness goals.

The 80/20 Rule in Nutrition

Eighty percent of your physical results will come from the food you put in your body. This concept can be very hard for some people. For some, it takes more discipline to eat right and avoid harmful foods than it does to exercise regularly. The most important things you do in life are often the most difficult, and the same is true for your physical objectives.

Highlight that last sentence, will ya?! Them is words to live by!

There are many ways you can apply the 80/20 rule to the way you eat. You don't have to live a tortured existence trying to maintain 100 percent perfection.

- Resolve to eat clean 80 percent of the time. You have to give yourself a little wiggle room. Okay, so 20 percent of the time you might not be eating from the highest tier, but you don't need to beat yourself up about it.

- Instead of *stuffing* yourself, give your stomach some time to digest your food by *stopping* yourself when you believe you're 80 percent full. Leave 20 percent of your stomach empty to help you digest and give your body time to catch up.

- Eighty percent of what you eat needs to be what you would feed an athlete (yeah, you!). In other words, a minimum of 80 percent of the time you should eat whole foods that fall within the ratios of the diet you've chosen for yourself (e.g., 40 percent protein, 30 percent carbs, 30 percent fat, or whatever formula works best for your goals and which can be sustained for the rest of your life).

- No more than 20 percent of the time should you eat outside of that target range. Set yourself up for success. Very few people can eat 100 percent clean, and they're easy to spot. (To be honest, they're not that fun to be around!)

- When you have to choose between nutrition and fitness, always make your nutrition a bigger priority. (Honestly, and not to add undue pressure, there are very few instances where you might have to choose. But let's just say that life chooses for you.)

Recently I had a flight scheduled for New York leaving at 9:00 a.m. from Los Angeles. This meant that to get through security for my flight, make the 1-hour drive to the airport, and still have time to shower and pick out a cute travel outfit, I'd need to be up and exercising by 4:45 a.m. at the latest. Of course I stayed up too late packing for the trip, and when my alarm sounded, I slept right through it! Luckily, Bret woke me up with enough time to still shower and make my flight, but I had missed my window of opportunity to exercise for the day.

Now, under most circumstances, this would have made me fuming mad. But instead, I reminded myself that considering the workout I had planned, the most I would have burned would have been around 400 calories. Instead of worrying, I reminded myself that just by eliminating 200 calories from my diet that day and

strolling through the airport terminal once I arrived, I would more than take care of the calories I missed in my workout. Heck, I could have even eaten those extra calories if I'd wanted to and simply added a little intensity to my workout the next day.

The 80/20 Rule in Fitness

Just because 80 percent of your results will come from your nutrition doesn't mean that you can or should neglect the 20 percent that is made up of your physical pursuits. In fact, I'd have to say that 80 percent of my positive attitude and energy level is due to my fitness pursuits! So keep in mind that exercise and fitness are important for a variety of reasons.

Additionally, for most people, regular exercise can make sticking to your healthy diet much easier. When you exercise, you have incentive to eat right!

Realize that exercise is an action that brings results. When it comes to your fitness, consistency is critical. It is too easy to let one day slip by, and then another. Before long, you're losing energy and confidence in your resolve. Force yourself, even if your workout is half the amount of time you planned to get in. Staying motivated, even when it's only a mini workout, helps keep you on track!

Plan to exercise 9 out of 10 days. When you do that, life will probably kidnap one of those days, but because you've allowed for these inevitabilities, you're still safely in the 80/20 range.

Always strive to give 100 percent to the workouts you do get to. Perfection isn't possible—or healthy, for that matter. We are human, and we have to live with other humans. Even if you are enough of a lunatic to achieve 100 percent adherence to an exercise program, there are other humans in your life who are not nearly as perfect, and they may have an effect on your workout schedule.

People make mistakes. You have to be forgiving (of yourself and others!) when errors happen. Expect that there will be emergencies, family needs, an illness, or that your body needs rest. You're creating a healthy and balanced life, not a scientifically perfect formula. Remember that the 80/20 rule is only a guideline.

So in business and productivity, focus on the top 20 percent, but in health and fitness, it's the 80 percent where you'll reap the greatest rewards!

Daily PUSH

1. Identify any item from your reverse-engineered brainstorm that might account for 80 percent of your momentum in the next month. Add it to your to-do list.

2. Schedule your workouts for the next 10 days, allowing just 1 scheduled day for rest and making mental arrangements to lose 1 day due to life's unexpected interruptions.

NOTES

_____

_____

_____

_____

_____

_____

_____

RANDOM Eating

Change Your Behavior and the Brain Will Follow!

Today we'll talk about the real reasons we're eating. Most of the time when we eat, it's not to satisfy our hunger but to change the way we feel.

Yes, I'm talking about what is usually described as "emotional eating." But let's stop using that term. For one thing, many people don't identify with it, especially if they don't consider themselves to be emotional people.

For another, the term "emotional eating" often conjures up the image of an overweight, middle-aged woman sobbing uncontrollably on her laundry- and feline-covered couch while devouring spoonful after spoonful of Ben & Jerry's. Oh sure, she's out there, but for most of us, it's not quite so dramatic.

For most of us, emotional eating is more an issue of mindless, unconscious eating—in other words, eating when we are neither hungry nor in need of nutrients. So let's call it *random eating!* Are you cool with that? Who can't relate to the concept of random eating?

The key to eliminating the habit of random eating is learning to identify what triggers it, redirecting our behavior, and better understanding why we eat just to eat.

I know you've been inundated with information on emotional eating. Today, I'll teach you how to identify the red flags of random eating and how to cope with and correct it.

Identify the Trigger

The first tool in your toolbox is your brain—specifically, the awareness you have when you "show up" for your own life. You can use that awareness to identify your food triggers.

Nine times out of 10, when we eat, it's not because we're hungry. It is because we're feeling something. Have you ever gotten a call from a family member, or a certain troublesome business associate or colleague, that raises your blood pressure? You *feel* your anxiety level creep up, you *feel* your stomach twist into a knot, and as soon as you hang up, your first instinct may be to eat.

Or maybe you've found yourself dead tired at the end of the day and you still have to fold laundry and empty the dishwasher before you can go to bed. At that moment, you feel an emotion. You long to be cared for. You need a break. You feel overworked and underappreciated. Feeling a bit sorry for yourself, you decide if no one else is going to take care of you, you'll treat yourself. And there you are, taking a quick break with a glass of wine or a big bowl of ice cream. "I really deserve this," you rationalize.

In these moments, as you turn to food or drink, you're feeling *something*, and you need to identify it. It may be anxiety, boredom, stress, or depression. You may feel tired, overwhelmed, nervous, or excited. You may even be procrastinating. Whatever it is, what you're *not* feeling, typically, is hunger. The key is to figure out what feelings are triggering your eating.

Get Aware

This process begins with an open-eyed look at *why* and *when* you find yourself just eating to eat.

I recently tapped into a common trigger for myself. I was at my computer, wading through a slew of e-mails.

Eating Doesn't Fix Problems—It Makes Them Worse

Interestingly, when we eat in response to a trigger, we do so in a manner that all but eliminates the joy of food. Snacks, meals, and even a food binge in response to a feeling can trigger the near equivalent of an alcoholic blackout. It's not uncommon at the end of the day to exclude that episode from your accounting of calories or food consumption. We have very little recollection and nearly zero satisfaction from random eating. It's as if it didn't happen.

When triggered by an experience, a feeling, an environment, or simply habit, turning to food doesn't fix the problem, not even for a minute. It only masks the feeling of confusion, boredom, sadness, etc. The good news is, once you recognize that food isn't the answer to your problems, you can start to change your mindless or emotional eating habits and begin to forge real change in your body and your life!

Most require only a quick, nearly mindless reply, "Got it! Thanks!" "Wednesday at noon works for me, too." Because I am a business owner with lots of employees, mixed in with the simple e-mails are always a few messages that require some problem solving. The next category of e-mails are those that give me what I call "brain pain." These might include complex problem solving, strategizing, heading off future problems, etc.

Said e-mail on this day was from one of our manufacturers explaining that even though we had just spent $50K on rush product delivery for a pending event, the shipment would not be arriving in time for said event. Um . . . WHAT??!?

Brain pain. Okay, there must be a solution, an alternative. My wheels begin to spin. I need to stop and think this one through.

Next, I slip into autopilot . . . Destination: kitchen (most days I work from home). My brain continues to sort through this as my eyes scan the fridge shelves, searching up and down for something to eat. I must be hungry. Nothing. I think to myself, "I need to go grocery shopping." Back to the problem at hand. "How am I going to get product produced for an event 2 weeks away?" I wander into the pantry. Aha! There it is! The solution to this prodigious dilemma . . . instant relief from my brain pain . . . something crunchy!

What I was feeling wasn't hunger. What I *was* feeling was a knot in my stomach and the stress of a rather complicated equation. In that moment, I realized that my random eating is often triggered when I have something tough to think through, a complex problem. It was a trigger to snack, a trigger to eat, a trigger to fix. My brain was telling me "you need to fix this" and

my behavior was to turn to the first and most comforting fix available, food.

Identifying that a cluttered mind is my random eating trigger gave me personal insight. When you have the presence of mind to understand why and when you do things, it gives you the power to change. I felt enlightened by this knowledge. I was learning something about myself I had never realized before. Oh sure, I have plenty of triggers that I'm aware of, but until that very moment, I had overlooked my "brain pain" e-mails.

Identifying what triggers your random eating is the most important skill in your quest to take control of your weight.

Take Action

To find an alternative behavior that replaces snacking, you must first identify what behaviors eliminate or help soothe the emotion or feeling that triggers your random eating episode. *Then* you can substitute the *feelings* for *behaviors* that actually provide relief.

So let's walk through this. What is your most common trigger? Write a few down or, at a minimum, put this book down for a moment, close your eyes, and really give it some thought. (Insert *Jeopardy!* theme music here.)

Is it a particular event, action, person, or memory that triggers an emotion for you? What is that emotion? Let's say that it's anger or even boredom that you're feeling. We know that random eating doesn't solve the issue that triggered you to feel that way, right? We agree so far? So what are our options? What actions can we take?

As I see it, there are three:

- Eat! This will help you to escape the feeling for a moment.

- Call a good therapist (or friend!) and get in a quick session on your way to the kitchen.

- Find an alternative behavior that also allows you to better cope with the feeling.

Look, I'm not here to offer you a Band-Aid. I suppose you're thinking the correct answer to the above is number 3. In most cases, you're right. However, if food has become your drug—and we're not talking about sneaking a few Hershey's Kisses but engaging in the kind of random eating or compulsive restricting of calories, that has taken over your life—then finding alternative behaviors will

Daily**PUSH**

1. Using pen and paper, create a brainstorm of the most common things you're feeling when you find yourself eating randomly.

2. Next, list the desired emotion or feeling that you would like to replace the undesirable feelings.

Example:
- ▶ Undesirable feeling = Anger, sadness
- ▶ Desired feeling = Joy, happiness

3. From the list you've created in response to step 2, create three or four activities that will help you achieve your desired emotion or feeling.

Example:
Alternate activities:
- ▶ Listen to my favorite playlist.
- ▶ Write a thank-you note to someone I appreciate.
- ▶ Call a friend to make plans for the weekend.

NOTES

_____

_____

_____

provide you with only a temporary solution.

But your *long-term* success is hinged on your commitment to get well. The experiences and early childhood traumas that led to food addiction can be just as addictive and destructive when they're transferred to an alternative behavior like compulsive exercise or even alcoholism.

Short term or long term, our goal is to learn that it's okay to feel. But sometimes that is best done with the help of a trained professional in a safe environment. So for right now, we're going to look at short-term solutions, but it's important for you to know this: The deeper and the scarier the "feeling" or emotion, the more important it is for you to seek long-term solutions. (Hello? Are you still there? If you just found yourself tuning me out in these last few sentences, it's probably because there's something in you that feels this is all too powerful to process. Ignore it. If I just busted you drifting off, that's impeding your success!)

Get the Feeling You Want from the Action That Provides It

Above, you identified the feeling that triggers your random eating. Let's say it's boredom. You eat not because you're hungry but because you're bored.

Now imagine the emotion you'd like to feel. If you're feeling boredom, your desired feeling might be excitement. In my own "brain pain" example above, the feeling was stress or confusion and my desired feeling was clarity and serenity.

Next, visualize what you would or could do to feel the desired emotion. If you want to feel excitement, what excites you that you can do in that moment? Skydiving on your lunch hour just might not be in the cards, but perhaps Googling a location where you might be able to do that is!

An intense solo workout clears my mind and makes me feel calm. Some people do yoga. I run. I don't run for speed but for clarity. What seems jumbled, insurmountable, and overwhelming as I lace up my running shoes is simple by the end of my run.

Exercise is one of the most effective ways to change your mood and provide relief from an uncomfortable feeling. But let's face it, it's not always feasible to drop everything and go for a brisk walk. That's why I want you to stop what you're doing right now and make a list of at least one non-exercise-related activity that gives you relief from your most common emotionally triggered random eating.

Important Person
PROMISE

Make Your Word Another
Weight-Loss Weapon

Today we're putting some real power behind both your Push and health goals. With just a few text messages and a minute or two of scrolling through your phone contacts, we'll put into effect one of the most powerful forms of accountability known to mankind.

But before we get to that, I want to tell you a true story about a real woman who did just what you have the opportunity to do today—if you dare. After you read about Meredith, I think you will.

Meredith's Story

In 2006, I was hosting a fitness camp in Orange County, California, with hundreds of fans and fitness enthusiasts from all over the country. On the second day of the camp, I asked the crowd for volunteers: those who might be brave enough to make the group a public promise.

A hand from near the back of the room rose timidly above the rest. Meredith, a woman clearly struggling with morbid obesity, stood up. With tears in her eyes and a quavering voice, she shared with us the courage she had to muster just to come to this camp.

Then she promised me and hundreds of

strangers that when she returned to camp next year, she'd be 100 pounds lighter.

She had come alone, didn't know a soul. She hadn't flown in years and wondered how she would fit in just one plane seat. She assumed she would be the heaviest person there. She wondered if she'd make it through a live workout. She worried she might be judged for her size and wouldn't be able to cope with being around so many fit people.

But once she landed and spent her first day with us, the courage she gained from overcoming her initial fears gave her the confidence to do more. Not the least of which was vocalizing such a commitment.

She later shared with me that she found my Turbo Jam program while watching late-night infomercials from her adjustable bed during a weight-related health-scare hospital stay. She made herself a promise to lose enough weight to make the trip to my Southern California camp to meet me in person. Needless to say, she followed through on that one.

But her latest commitment, her new promise, was now public.

She asked if I had any advice to help her reach her 100-pound goal in 12 months. I explained to her that she was going to lose 5 pounds at a time. Focus on what she must do first and keep herself accountable. She had tears running down her face, but I could see a familiar look in her eyes. It's the look that people get when they have "flipped the switch."

I asked her to make me a promise: She would e-mail me each time she had checked "lose 5 pounds" from her list. Let's just say I heard from her *often* in 2006.

In 2007, she returned to my camp having exceeded her goal. She had lost 117 pounds. Not only had she lost the weight, but thanks to the help and motivation of others, she went on to become a fitness instructor and had even taught her first class, all in the span of a year.

Never underestimate the power of accountability and a public promise.

The Power of a Promise

When you make a promise, you stick to it. The words *I promise* are so incredibly powerful that we will rarely speak them unless we are 100 percent positive the outcome is within our control. We can deliver!

And we don't make promises we can't keep. For example, when my daughter asks if her pug, Studley, will live forever, I can't make that promise because I personally cannot make that happen. I can promise her, however, that Studley will live a very full and happy life.

Promises are public commitments made when we know we have the personal power to deliver. In fact, the only variable is your determination and discipline, both of which you fortify by making said promise. When you vow to do something, you have given your word. Your word is like placing a lien against your own integrity. If you want your integrity (and who doesn't?), you need to deliver on your promise! We all feel an overwhelming responsibility to follow through when we give someone our word.

By making your Push goal and health goal promises (and yes, it's quite likely you will be making promises to more than one person today), you reinforce your commitment and establish a heavy-duty layer of accountability.

A promise to yourself is very nice, but let's be honest—it's easier to break a promise to yourself than it is to break a sweat. If we can't change the fact that when we make ourselves a promise we often break it, then let's work with what we know *does* work: making a promise to someone else!

Most of us have conditioned ourselves to take care of everyone else first and place our own needs last. We crave acceptance. We long for the approval and admiration of others. So when another person is counting on us, come hell or high water, we will do absolutely everything in our power to avoid breaking a promise or letting someone down to whom we have given our word.

Don't get me wrong! It's certainly a wonderful human trait to place the needs of others before our own. I believe, however, it is one of the reasons why so many people end up sidetracked from their own hopes and dreams. You would never dream of breaking a promise to a significant person in your life. But you wouldn't hesitate to break a promise you had made to yourself if it meant doing something for someone else.

When you give your word to someone, you become personally, emotionally, and ethically committed to achievement.

Prep Work for Your Daily Push: Pick Your Important People

Today's assignment is to take your Push goal and your health goal and turn them into two separate promises. Grab a pencil and let's do this together.

1. Write your Push goal at the top of the left-hand side of the form below. You'll write your health goal on the right-hand side. Just below those headings, you'll see several blank lines for you to fill in.

On each of those blank lines, list the names of the people whom the achievement of your Push goal will most positively affect. Now, it doesn't have to be life-shattering to them, but I do want you to come up with a few folks who will feel your impact.

For example, when I set a Push goal for myself to teach 100,000 people how to set priorities, goals, and master their to-do list with my 30-Day Challenge, I made a public promise to my agent, my husband, my IT department, my Facebook fans, my Twitter followers, and just about anyone else I knew would hold me to it.

2. Under your health goal, I want you to do the same thing. Who are the people you'd rather cut off your own arm than disappoint? Add these people to your list. To promise your young children that you will quit smoking is a fantastic idea, but I would also add your employer, your best friend, your friends who smoke, the liquor store clerk where you buy your cigs, and anyone else to whom you know this might matter.

Before we're done making that list of "promise people," give it another glance.

I want you to include any important person in your life whose opinion you greatly value—a person you'd be mortified to let down. The more people you put on this list, the better.

I need you to make sure you call, text, e-mail (whatever your favorite mode of communication) the people on your list and let them know you're making them a promise. Promise them that you're going to achieve your Push goal in the next 12 months. Give them your word and do it right now.

Follow the instructions on the opposite page. This must be done today, no excuses. Do this before anything else. It will only take a few seconds.

1. Use your preferred mode of communication to call, text, e-mail, Facebook, and instant message the important people on your list and let them know what promise you're making.

2. Explain why you've made this promise to them and extend permission to them to help keep you on track.

PUSH GOAL

_____

List of people

_____

_____

_____

_____

_____

HEALTH GOAL

_____

List of people

_____

_____

_____

_____

_____

This is your very first task of the day. It will take only a few minutes.

Go Public with Your Promises

There's nothing worse than a politician who fails to follow through on a promise made on national television during campaign months. When Domino's Pizza was blasted after two of its employees posted a YouTube video depicting ingredients falling on the floor and other disgusting things happening to your "pie" before the delivery guy knocks on the door, the CEO of the company took to the airwaves and promised Domino's customers that there would be some big changes. He promised to improve the quality of the pizza and restore consumers' faith in their product. Domino's delivered.

Politicians are notorious for breaking promises. People of integrity, on the other hand, make public promises to restore faith in their word, to assure their greatest supporters that they won't let them down. To make a promise public to the world is an act of bravery. It says you believe in yourself 100 percent and you're willing to stake your integrity.

I want you to make your promise public (assuming that it's not too personal). I want you to post your promise on your Facebook page! Post it everywhere! Make a YouTube video, tweet it, Skype it, have a live Ustream.tv broadcast. Make your promise public to your friends, your family, and all of your co-workers. Make this promise to the universe.

I know you feel the momentum of your success and your new habits building energy. Success is your destiny. Today's assignment is about making that Push goal a *promise*. And you will be able to keep your promise to the universe, not because you've closed your eyes and dreamed about it, not because you made a vision board or a list of 10 goals. You are destined to achieve your Push goal and your health goal because you have the foundation! You have a plan! You have a system in place and people in your life for whom you will push!

DAY 24
Fat-Free FRIENDS

Hang with Positive Peeps Who Won't Weigh You Down

You are the average of the five people you
spend the most time with.

—Jim Rohn

Don't worry, I'm not going to ask you to find a bunch of super-
models to hang out with. When I say fat-free friends, I mean,
drama-free, healthy, supportive, successful types.

Today, we're going to work on a plan to help you tune in to why you choose to spend time and focus on certain people and how to develop stronger relationships with healthier people.

To a great extent, the people you spend your focus and energy on influence who you are, how you view yourself, and the person you will become. When I think of fat, I think of a gooey, unattractive substance that sticks to the bones, weighs me down, and makes me slow, lethargic, and unhappy. We all have people in our lives who can make us feel this way. Today's objective is to heighten your sense of success. Your sense of success is much like your sense of smell or your sense of sight. Tapping into your sense of success will help you evaluate your circle of influence (those people you devote the most energy to) and decide if it's time to make some changes.

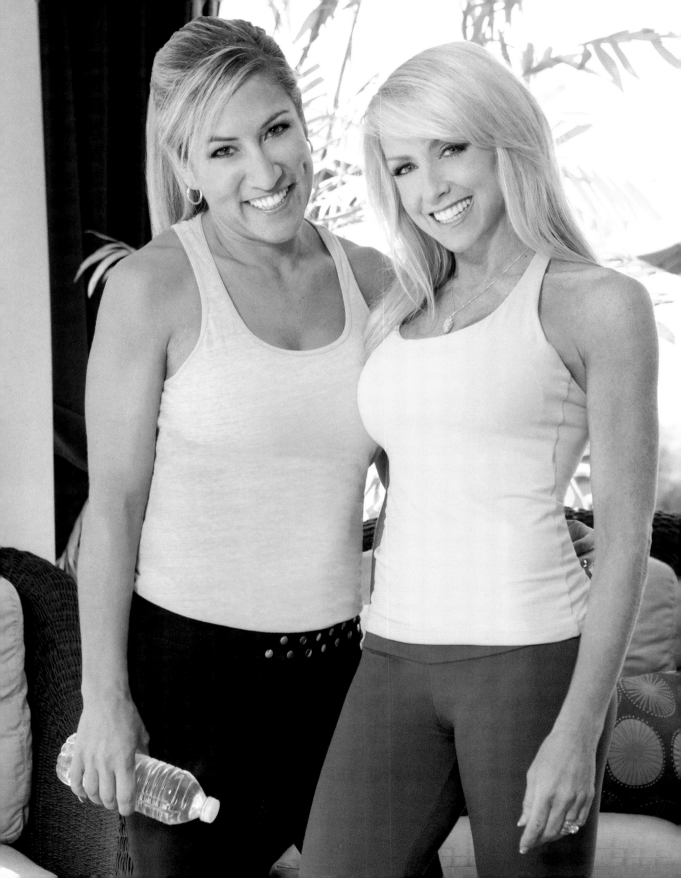

Detaching from Success Suckers

Energy vampires, Debbie downers, success suckers—call 'em what you may, but don't call them part of your success equation. Perhaps up to this point you have thought of some of these folks as friends, maybe as your charity case friends. Now I ask you to take this journey seriously and realize these people are friendly acquaintances but not necessarily quality friends.

When you're mindful of your sense of success, you will be keenly aware that you are investing time with the wrong people. One way of knowing is to ask yourself honestly if you feel, well, the superior human in their company. Ouch. Now I don't mean that you're taller or cuter. I mean to say that you know you have it going on and you know they do not and probably never will have their sh#@ together. Their poor choices and bad habits help you to feel better about your own. Their mediocrity makes you feel like a mover and a shaker. Not easy to admit, but critically important for you to be mindful of.

Sometimes the people who weigh us down do so by holding us hostage on a hamster wheel. Desperate to impress, you run on that wheel faster and faster in a feverish effort to win their favor. Only that wheel leads to nowhere and nothing . . . except exhaustion. Winning their approval is impossible, as they're not happy with themselves. They don't really want you to succeed, and they're really bothered when good things happen for you. Perhaps it's jealousy, insecurity, or their own hurt. The impossible feat of winning their favor leaves you depleted of energy and confidence. Ironically, the last thing in the world this type of person wants for you is your long-term success. You are most useful to them as a subordinate friend. Think over this description. Does someone come to mind?

Wounded Bird Collectors

Once a year my company, Powder Blue Productions, holds auditions for new presenters. We look for leaders in the community, those who find joy in helping others succeed. They are naturally positive people who intuitively mentor others to outshine them. They teach fitness enthusiasts how to become fitness instructors and wellness leaders. In addition to examining their résumés, experience, and audition tapes demonstrating their teaching and speaking skills, we also profile their personalities. From time to time, we find a nearly perfect candidate. The only downside is that this person sometimes turns out to be what I call a "wounded bird collector."

When I was a kid, we lived for many years out in the country in a quiet farm town in the center of Michigan. The walk from the bus stop to our front door was miles and miles down dusty dirt roads. (My mother swears it was only about 100 yards.) But on those long walks home, I would often spot a dying bird on the side of the road.

Ever the optimist, I would scoop up the broken-winged robin with a missing eye, carry him in my pocket the rest of the way home, and place him in my makeshift trauma center: a grass-lined shoe box. Through the night, I would make sure he was warm and nurse my tiny patient back to health on a diet of watered-down Cream of Wheat cereal. I'd speak sweetly to him. "You're gonna make it, little guy!"

They never did. I buried a lot of shoe boxes before I eventually realized that what I should be looking for was a healthy bird, a bird that actually had a shot at survival. (And, yes, to this day, I have several parrots!)

Wounded bird collectors are kindhearted, caring folks who have a soft spot for the weak. They possess all the leadership qualities we look for, but their sense of success is slightly askew. These individuals often help and mentor, but they surround themselves with people who are so broken, so negative, so damaged, that their own journey to success is, well, to put it mildly, something that's many therapy sessions away.

Now listen, before you go calling me a cold-hearted bee-otch who doesn't see the value in everyone, let me explain. There's a difference between helping those in need and surrounding yourself with people so broken you become distracted from the work you need to do yourself.

In our many years of working with leaders, we have learned that the people candidates associate themselves with is a strong indicator of the candidates' self-image.

Everyone deserves a chance. Your past does not define you. Only where you're headed is what matters. Maintaining your friendships with people unwilling to move themselves forward, who are relying on you to lift them up and shuffle their feet along, is only hurting both of you. If your friend is not taking action, not moving in the right direction, even at a snail's pace, carrying this friend is not going to help. It's time to ask yourself how it serves you to spend so much time trying to put this person's life back on track. It might be because there's no time to work on yourself when you're so busy being noble.

Opposites Attract

You've heard that positive people attract positive people. But it is also true that opposites attract. I believe this is valuable in business relationships, partnerships, and to some extent in marriage. However, as it pertains to friends, work to fill your five favorite people spots with the names of those who share your positive nature.

Positive energy is your priceless life force. You can't afford to allow success suckers to empty your account. People who start every conversation with an excuse and a complaint do so because it benefits them. They get your attention. It's become part of who they are. They believe they themselves have little of interest, so they often start with a complaint or their own personal drama.

Choose Wisely

Not much you can do now to pick different parents. (Simma down, Mom, you know I'm just making a point!) As for friends, you've got choice. Make a decision in your mind—not on Facebook: With whom do you want to work to invest more? This is a little "note to self."

I do not recommend you share your selections with anyone else. It's too easy for your thinking to be misconstrued. You don't need to schedule a "Hey, yeah, um, by the way, we're not friends anymore" conversation. Simply decide to invest less time. You're a kind person, and you certainly see all of a person's great qualities, so of course you'll always be friendly. You'll just become more aware of not investing time with someone who doesn't lift you up.

What Do Fat-Free Friends Look Like?

I can't tell you what they look like, but I can share some personality traits to help you spot them!

1. They're readers. Fat-free friends want to know more and learn as much as they can. They're curious. They find other people interesting and want to know more. They want to know how successful people do what they do. They read about success and study the great habits of others.

2. They share. Fat-free friends want the world for you, and they share in your joy when you reach your goals. They share their experiences and knowledge. They are informal teachers and coaches.

3. They hang around with other successful folks. The kind of friends you should spend more time with hang with other successful folks. They find inspiration in others. They're attracted to friends who lift others.

4. They call you out when you are taking the easy route on the wrong path. They want you to be the very best version of yourself and won't tolerate it when you are doing things that are harmful, hurtful, or dangerous.

Change Is Growth. Growth Is Good

Letting go, even when you know someone isn't good for you, can be difficult. We fear change because the status quo represents comfort. But good things happen when you're willing to get a little uncomfortable.

Letting go of people who don't carry genuine love in their heart for you is something you can do for yourself. These people's negative nature has nothing to do with you. How they have treated your relationship or their own potential says more about them than it does about you.

It's not personal. It's about them. Someone who gossips and puts other people down in your presence is doing the same about you when you're not around.

Be Selective

There are six billion people on the planet. Pick your friends carefully. Don't you dare say you don't know many positive, successful people. You do. Open your eyes and take a look around you. If you don't see anyone, attract those people into your life with your new attitude. Invest your most valuable asset (time) with those who bring out the best in you and not those who are looking for a buddy to make them feel comfortable with their own unhealthy choices.

Set clear measures. Do the people you select . . .

- Support your vision for a healthy successful life?
- Lift you up and keep you accountable?
- Have a positive influence on who you are?
- Have respect for themselves, their relationships, their health and fitness?

Do you aspire to have some of the positive character traits of this individual?

Daily **PUSH**

1. What is the kind of person do you want your friends to hold you accountable to be?

2. What five friends do you spend the most time with currently?

3. On a scale of 1 to 10 (1 = not so much and 10 = totally!), give each person a ranking base on how well they align with how you've described yourself in point 1.

4. List one to five acquaintances that embody the characteristics you desire in yourself.

5. Add reaching out to each person you've listed in point 4 to your to-do list. Begin building those relationships today.

NOTES

_____

_____

_____

_____

_____

A friend who is funny or beautiful or outgoing or who consoles you when you make a bad decision is certainly not necessarily someone who makes you a better person. Relationships should be mutually beneficial. Notice I didn't say they should be equally beneficial. If you're expecting equality in relationships, you've landed on the wrong planet. Every relationship has one person who does more than the other party. Just make sure you don't have resentment over that imbalance.

Positive energy is your priceless life force. Protect it. Don't allow people to draw from your reserves; select friends who recharge your energies.

Always Play Up

A few years ago, my husband (who happens to be a coach) suggested that my son play on a basketball team where the boys were a year or two older. I said to my husband, "Why would we do that? You know he's going to sit on the bench. That doesn't seem productive." He said, "When you play up, your teammates are better, older, stronger, and more experienced than you. You don't want to let them down, so you rise to their level."

Play up. I'm not asking you to cut people out of your life, but I am asking you to invest your time with people will push you to be your best. Winners love to see other people win.

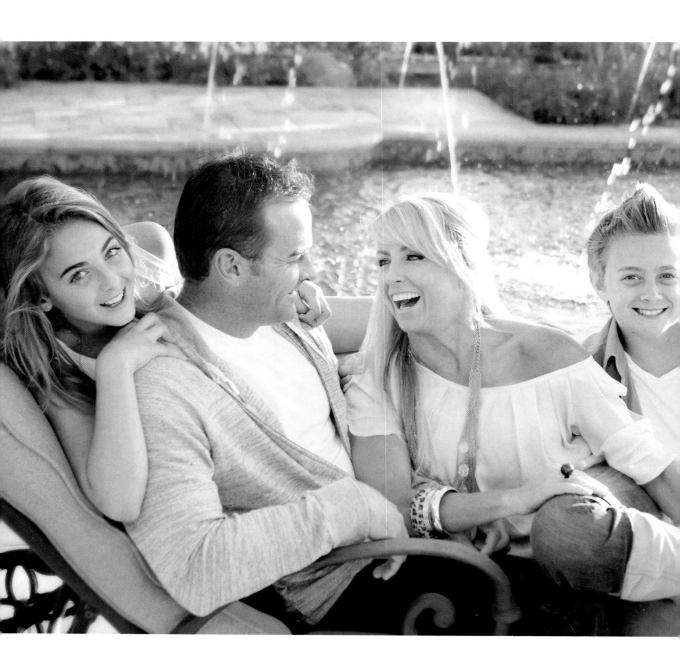

Give Your Relationship(s) a MAKEOVER

Loving Yourself While Giving Your All

"Love is the basic need of human nature,
for without it, life is disrupted emotionally,
mentally, spiritually and physically."

—Dr. Karl Menninger

Does it really matter if you're a size 0 if you have discord in your most important relationships? If having a ripped six-pack meant driving a wedge between you and your spouse, would you still pursue it? I hope the answer is no.

When people lose weight and change their habits, their lifestyle changes, their confidence increases, and relationships are affected.

Lasting weight loss means teaming a new way of thinking about yourself with a change in your lifestyle. Inevitably, you will form new friendships, tastes, habits, and patterns.

As people develop new lives, it's not uncommon for their partners to feel lonely, left behind, angry, resentful, abandoned, and maybe even jealous. Today I ask you to break away from your own success, your own healing, and your own journey so that you can recognize the importance of having your partner by your side. I'll also share with you some simple habits that will strengthen your partnership and fortify your journey together as a team.

I've sought to understand the difference between those couples who grow stronger and those who grow apart. The difference boils down to making a decision to do more than your part, more than you think is fair. The difference boils down to one overriding principle: Love and support is more important than skinny jeans. But with a little extra work, both can be yours!

Could Your Bangin' Body Test Your Love?

Before we go further, keep in mind two guiding principles:

1. Every romantic partner wants to feel important, like the center of your universe.

2. Any disconnect your partner is feeling at this stage has to do with fear. This fear or anxiety can be caused by a disruption in the balance of your attention, conspicuous rise in your happiness, and your newfound confidence.

That last point might not make sense to you at first. Seriously, why would your partner not be happy about all this positive change?

Because the shift in your mind-set and redirected attention might lead your partner to believe he or she now has lost significance in your world.

In the mind of the person experiencing this physical and emotional transformation (you), it gradually becomes clear you want no part of your old ways. Your thinking has changed along with your view of yourself. Realize it or not, you've become fiercely protective of your new you.

But your partner, even if he or she is supportive of your new healthy habits, hasn't been clued in on emotional nature of this transformation. It's still business as usual. No one has handed out notes on your recent game change.

Distance, resentment, jealousy, and fear are just a few of the emotions felt by someone whose partner experiences a rather dramatic change in lifestyle or physical appearance. Your partner might feel threatened by this unavoidable change or shift in the relationship, or feel judged for not making the same changes, and may purposely or inadvertently find ways to sabotage your progress or belittle your success.

A partner suddenly no longer feels like the center of that person's universe. The newly fit and happy partner begins to derive joy from within instead of from food or from exclusively catering to the needs of others. The newly fit may even feel a lack of connection to a partner who has no interest in or who is threatened by the changes.

The resentment and distance continue to build. Neither partner may realize this is going on, but both begin to feel the disconnect. Each waits for the other to take a step closer; however, in doing so, they are walking farther and farther apart.

Before long, you're doing everything as individuals and less as a couple. You have your activities and your partner has his or her own—different friends, different schedules, different food, and different habits. The bond weakens. The resentment grows.

It's no one's fault, but someone needs to step up and be the hero. And it needs to be you. The good news is, if you're aware of the signs of discontent and arm yourself with a plan of action, your partnership can actually flourish and become stronger than ever.

The first step? Reexamining your relationship—and getting gut-wrenchingly honest.

Own Your Part of the Problem— And Solve It!

Fitness and weight are far deeper than just finding a great exercise program or eating less. I'm not speaking as an expert or therapist. I'm coming from 20 years of experience as a fitness coach and 16 years of marriage—nearly 20 years with the same partner (my darling husband, Bret).

A person who has let him- or herself go, has low energy and low self-esteem, and who has been dealing with the stigma associated with being overweight has more to deal with than simply shedding some pounds. If you have allowed yourself to gain weight to the point that you don't identify with the person in the mirror,

you have probably also come to expect that people, even your spouse, will treat you as "less than worthy" of respect, care, love, and kindness.

Often, when I meet people at the beginning their fitness journey, they have allowed themselves to slip into last place on their list of importance. They have taught others to ignore them. They have taken care of everyone and everything else and practiced a great deal of self-loathing.

When people don't like themselves, they don't expect much from others. The way you feel about yourself affects the dynamics in every relationship you have.

When someone begins to look and feel better, self-esteem naturally rises. For the first time in a long time, you might be looking in the mirror and thinking, "I'm looking good. I'm feeling good. I can do this." You begin to recognize your potential. You're the same person you've always been, but lately you've begun to believe you deserve better.

This is where things can get treacherous!

Before long, you may choose to move from acceptance of poor behavior to resentment. Now you realize you have allowed friends, family members, partners, even co-workers to treat you in a certain way, and it's not cool. It's like you've suddenly come to your senses. You're awake! And it feels like you're being inauthentic to yourself to allow this treatment to continue.

Notice the word *choose* in the last paragraph. How you feel about others is a choice. Your mind-set, your attitude in this process is critical. Allow negative thoughts about someone in your life to build, and before long that person becomes the villain. You can't recall a moment of happiness. Your anger grows. You honestly believe you have no personal culpability. It's the other person's fault. You just aren't willing to take it anymore.

Hold the arms of your chair for a moment . . . I'm about to push you: You are just as much to blame as your partner, maybe more.

You are also the person capable of improving your marriage. I know you've been told that a partnership is 50/50. And those who subscribe to that way of thinking are likely to be in the 50 percent statistic whose marriage ends in divorce.

Life is not fair. Partnerships are not fair. You are 100 percent responsible for both, and when you believe that, and operate that way, your relationship will thrive.

Loving Yourself, Saving Your Relationships

Here's the deal: As your body and habits have been changing, so too has your view of who you are and what you believe you deserve. And you know what? You *do* deserve better! And the best is yours to be had, but not at the expense of your relationships.

Slow your roll! Calm down! Stop feeling sorry for yourself and do this the right way. You can't change the rules overnight! You can't wake up one day and suddenly proclaim that you won't tolerate what you've been tolerating for years. That will get you exactly nowhere!

Here's an idea: Figure out what it is you want, what it is you deserve, and how you expect to get that.

Getting to where you want to be in your important relationships is a delicate dance. It begins by making your spouse or partner feel adored, even when you don't—at this moment anyway—think the world of that person.

You will.

You've got plenty of choices, but only one results in getting the two of you on the same page. All it takes is checking your ego at the door. Be the bigger person. This journey has been about becoming a better you. Why not be the humble hero to this relationship? True, there will be no trophy ceremony, but what reward could be better than a stronger relationship? With persistence, you can enjoy the happiness you both deserve.

You often hear "it takes two," but I think a more useful comment is "it takes one." In every relationship, one partner is more emotionally mature than the other. That's the way life is. It takes one partner willing to do more than his or her share. If that has to be you, so what! Do it.

Doing more than your share emotionally doesn't mean one partner is better or even cares more than the other. It means you are willing to swallow your pride, set aside the hurt, and make it work. It takes one person willing to grab the wheel and steer the ship with persistence and devotion. Not overnight, but before long your feelings will follow, and so too will your partner's.

And when weeks and months of consistently treating your partner as the center of your universe seems to have little or no effect, then move on to plan B. It may take some gentle, well-timed convincing, but one person should schedule time with a highly recommended therapist. If the first therapist you meet with doesn't help, that professional wasn't a good fit. Find another!

Six Keys to a Rock-Solid Bond

I'm not one of those people who doesn't believe in divorce. In fact, if there are no kids involved, I don't have much of an opinion. I just know that people are happier, kinder, nicer, and healthier when their relationships are strong and when they feel safe, protected, and loved by their partner. Strong relationships don't happen by accident. They take work—a lot more than most people think.

Let's assume, however, that you have a genuinely supportive partner excited about sharing this success journey with you. What can you do to strengthen your relationship?

EXPRESS GRATITUDE EVERY DAY Your most important habits are practiced daily. Expressing your sincere gratitude to your partner every day is perhaps one of the most impactful things you can do for your relationship.

Everyone longs to feel needed. So thank him or her for any small part in helping or supporting your journey. Try thank-yous like these:

- "It means a lot to me that you do things like caring for the kids so that I can fit a workout into my day."

- "It really helps when as a family we pick restaurants that have healthy options."

- "Thanks for understanding how important it is for me to create my to-do list every day."

Gratitude is important, and important tasks should be included on your to-do list and not left to chance. You might also write yourself a reminder on a stickie note.

DO DAILY "QUICK CONNECTS" Did you know you can improve communication without having to officially talk about it? The key to any relationship isn't necessarily a long, deep conversation where the two of you lay your feelings out on the table, but rather a connection. By the time "the talk" is necessary, you've missed out on many opportunities to connect.

A "connect" is any intentional attempt to remind partners of their importance: a text asking how their day is going, a handwritten note left in the car, a card, a surprise hug, a quick voice mail letting your partner know how much they mean to you or just that you're thinking of them. Think of each connection as a deposit into your "love bank." I know that sounds cheesy, but it's true. And it takes 100 deposits to balance just one withdrawal.

TELL THEM THINGS HAVE CHANGED— RESPECTFULLY If you're feeling differently about yourself and ready to ask for better treatment from others, then communicate your needs calmly, with sweetness and understanding, when the time is right.

Remember, it's you who has suddenly decided that what was okay before is no longer okay. You have the responsibility to ask your partner to help you with this transition. Finger-pointing and shouting "you . . . you . . . you" will only leave your partner feeling alienated, confused, and attacked. You can't expect anyone to read your mind. Lose your resentment and put yourself in the other person's shoes. Have this conversation slowly, over a period of time, and before you've built up the resentment that prevents many couples from repairing their relationship. What's the point of getting fit if you're all alone?!?

GET ON THE SAME PATH Partners walking down separate paths can't expect to stay together for long. If you want to be together forever, find a way to spend more time together. When it comes to work and exercise, it is the quality of the time spent. When it comes to your relationships, the quality is further enhanced by the quantity of time. Take extra steps to create an opportunity to do things together.

Think of the couples you know how have been happily married for 30, 40, even 50 years. I bet when you picture them, you picture them together. They share the same hobbies, friends, and mutual interests. Invite your partner to join you in your workouts. Should he or she decline, find another way to suggest spending time

Daily PUSH

1. Set a daily reminder on your to-do list to express gratitude toward your partner.

2. Decide on one weekly activity you will give up to spend that time with your partner.

NOTES

_____

_____

_____

_____

_____

_____

_____

_____

together. Work to help your spouse find a soul-mate workout. No one wants to be told what to do or that he or she "needs" to exercise. Be creative. Explain how much it would mean to you to be on this journey together. Go out of your way to make together-time happen.

DON'T SPEND TIME ALONE WITH OPPOSITE-SEX "FRIENDS" I'm going out on a limb here and say I'm sure many of you will disagree. This is a personal rule for Bret and me, and it's based on the practices of our own parents, each of whom are still married to the same people after 40-plus years! No friends of the opposite sex, unless it's a friend we both share, and time spent together is spent as a couple with this person, no alone time (no matter how perfectly innocent). Don't flirt with friends of the opposite sex. Respect your spouse by avoiding any situation that could be deemed uncomfortable. Avoid working out with friends of the opposite sex, unless of course your friend is gay! (Oh no, she didn't . . . Oh yes, I did!)

Why engage in activities that could potentially damage your relationship? Seems kinda silly. These marital guidelines are our own, and of course, there are exceptions to every relationship. Neither Bret nor I is the jealous type, but we've witnessed so many couples starting innocently with a night out with friends once a month, then once a week, then separate trips, and before we knew it, our friends were divorced.

I'm not suggesting time apart will lead to divorce. I am, however, suggesting that more time *together* will lead to a stronger relationship. This rule works well for our marriage. If you're married, the risks of spending time with someone of the opposite sex far outweigh the benefits. Why go there?

THINK OF THE KIDS I recently had a conversation with a student going through a divorce. She told me she would do anything for her three children, including dying for them.

And yet, when I pushed her to try a new counselor, she explained that she just couldn't bear to spend another month with her husband. If you say you would do anything for your children, then do everything you can to repair your marriage before deciding it's beyond healing. Have an open mind to the thought of falling in love again. Your history is the past. Your mindset is everything. Many studies show a direct correlation between childhood obesity rates and children from divorced families.

Those of us with young children have a far greater responsibility to the world to keep our marriages strong. The healthiest thing you can do for your kids is to strengthen your marriage. As a society, if we spent as much time and money working on our marriages as we did working on weight loss, the world would be a much better place. That's all.

Please know that I'm speaking to those of you who have a choice. Some do not. Ultimately, you must protect your children, and a volatile, unhealthy home is the worst place for a child. I can't help but put my arms around those of you who have endured the painful loss of a marriage and the guilt and hardship that so many parents experience when circumstances are simply out of your control. My heart goes out to you. But blame and self-loathing will not help your children. Not every marriage or relationship is in the best interest of the children. To raise healthy, strong, confident, and loving children, you must exemplify those qualities.

Curing the DISEASE to PLEASE

In 140 Characters or Fewer

Today you will have an aha moment. You'll read the lesson, walk to the closest mirror, look yourself directly in the eyes, smack yourself upside the head, smile, and say, "Duh!"

Today you'll memorize one simple phrase to successfully manage and *eventually* cure your disease to please.

I'm revealing this to the world, at the risk of tipping off all the people in my inbox with whom I've just used this reply. I have an obligation to share it, *because it works*. (Get out your highlighter, digital or physical!)

When somebody asks me to do something, anything . . . I respond with what I call the Golden Reply:

Thank you so much for thinking of me. Let me check my schedule and I'll get back to you.

Read it again: *Thank you so much for thinking*

of me. Let me check my schedule and I'll get back to you.

Duh! Right? The Golden Reply, or TGR, is so simple, so gracious—and so effective—you can't believe you hadn't mastered it earlier!

Don't get me wrong. Sometimes it makes sense to say, "I'll do that for you!" Certainly if my BFF needs frozen yogurt in the middle of the night, I'm there!

But you've got to learn the rules to the yes-or-no game. Once I got in the habit of using TGR, it helped me get over my fear that the person I was responding to would think I was a jerk. Now I'm able to gain a little wiggle room, check my commitments, and evaluate if saying yes makes sense. When I'm still not 100 percent sure, I review my posted list of priorities. Once I've looked at my priorities, my decision, whether yes or no, is made with confidence.

Finding a cure to my disease to please has allowed me to be significantly more productive—and it will help you, too. When you value your time, you honor your priorities and your commitment to live the life that you deserve. That's why today you'll learn to use TGR instead of the automatic default to yes.

Your New Favorite Phrase

So why didn't I just advise you to just use that one little word *no?* Because I'm a realist, and I'm not going to force you to say the word you're most afraid of. I also happen to have formerly suffered from the same crippling disease you may have: people pleasing. I understand that suggesting that a people pleaser "just say no" is like telling an alcoholic "just stop drinking" or an overeater to "just eat in moderation." Good luck with that.

You see, part of the reason why your people-pleasing disease has progressed to this level is because you are a doer! You're the one everyone counts on to get things done because others have come to expect that you'll do it. You make the time and ensure you get things done—for other people. The challenge is learning to do so in doses that allow you to get things done *for you, too*—and most important, to be successful and happy.

If all you do is take care of other people, they begin to make sure you're very busy doing just that. You stop making time for yourself. After a while, you're no longer doing things because you *want* to but rather because you feel a sense of self-imposed guilt.

You're convinced that someone, someday, is going to throw a parade in your honor for your selflessness. (I've picked out an outfit to wear on the float just in case they ever decide to put a parade together for me!) But the parade isn't coming. With the best of intentions, you've trapped yourself in your own makings, doing "things" to be liked and accepted.

When you learn to make this reply a habit, you get the distance and time you need to realistically evaluate the situation as well as your true motivation. Why are you considering saying yes? Is it because it feels good? Is it because it fits with your priorities and goals, or is it because you want the mean girl to like you?

My friend Lorie Marrero, author of *The Clutter Diet*, suggests the practice of donating a bag of clothes from your closet each time you return from the mall with a new bag of swag! Taking a cue from this fine advice, I suggest that each time you say *yes* to someone or something, balance your plate by saying *no* and eliminating something else. When you take on something new, you really need to release something else.

So the next time you're about to volunteer yourself to be the party planner, chauffeur your neighbor to Walmart three towns away, host a party to sell your friends a bunch of kitchen gadgets, or coordinate a project, consider what you could do with those hours. Oh sure, it might take only 2 or 3 hours this week, but can you imagine if you had those hours to devote to preparing healthy meals, trying a new workout, or working on your Push goal? Hello!

As a rule of thumb, do things for other people when it feels good, it makes sense, you're not currently overwhelmed, and it doesn't compromise your priorities. Ask yourself: "Is this the best use of my time?"

Sometimes the answer is yes. Zig Ziglar, success expert, is well known for saying, "You can have everything in life you want if you will just help enough other people get what they want." Doing for others is noble, selfless, and rewarding—in moderation. But everyone defines "moderation" differently, and you've got to know what it means to you. When you so, so will everyone else.

Is Saying Yes Masking Your Fear of Failure?

Sometimes we enjoy "doing" for others so we can put off what we know we need to do for ourselves.

Anne, a graduate of one of my productivity programs, posted this note to me on Facebook.

Chalene, I need your help! About 2 years ago I lost 50 pounds with Turbo Kick. But over the course of the last year, I've gained most of that back. I know it's due to stress. You see, we have four children and live in an area where the cost of living is almost unbearable. My husband works for the government on a fixed income, which was substantially reduced last year. Even though we have cut back on almost everything, with his change of pay and because my kids are at an age where sports are getting very expensive, we are in a nightmare of a financial situation. We are losing our home and have maxed out every credit card. I volunteer at the kids' school 5 days a week. By the time I get home, dinner prepared, laundry started, and homework signed off on, the last thing in the world I want to do is exercise. I just don't have the energy to do it mentally or physically.

Am I crazy or is that simply *radonkulous??* By her own admission, her family is flat broke, risking the loss of their home, and she's "volunteering"

Warning!

Do not teach the Golden Reply to your children or staff. When reminded to pick up "dog bombs" early this week, my daughter, Cierra, was quick to reply, *"Thank you so much for thinking of me. Let me check my schedule and I'll get back to you."*

5 days a week? Hello? Earth to Mother Teresa!

I don't mean to make light of the situation. I love her for helping out at the school. Lord knows I volunteer my share of hours at the kids' school every year, and have done so since Brock was in kindergarten. But last year, while I was writing this book and had a few new projects on my plate, in order to be available for my own kids after 2:30 p.m. I had to cut back on my volunteer hours. (Oh, and while I'm thinking of it, our teachers are not paid enough to do what they do! You're all saints! Saints, I tell you!)

But there comes a point when you just need to get real. During a time of personal crisis, saying yes to extras is simply not an alternative. Do what you need to do for your family first. Volunteering your time is a selfless act *when the needs of your immediate family have been met*. Doing for others to avoid your own responsibilities is irresponsible.

We exchanged messages back and forth. I pushed Anne to consider a number of alternatives to improve her situation. I urged her to find part-time work during school hours. When she came up with 100 reasons why she would never find work, I then suggested she cut her volunteer hours in half and use that time to handle household responsibilities that were exhausting her at night, even consider exercising during those hours to help improve her mood, her outlook, and her energy level. Despite loads of opportunity to use that time to supplement her family's income, Anne was using her disease to please as an excuse to avoid doing what was difficult but which in the long run would best serve her family. You see, it's Anne's fear of failing that motivates her to say yes to things that really have little impact on her family's well-being. Anne's fear of failure becomes the roadblock to her success.

Know Your Motivation

Misplaced guilt is not a valid basis to take on more. Don't fall prey to the manipulation of those (well-conditioned family and friends) who have a great deal at stake when it comes to your disease! You know how when you make a really weird high-pitched noise around dogs, they quick-cock their heads and perk up their ears, as though a thought bubble above their heads would read "Hmmmmm?" Well, that's the reaction you'll get the first time you tell one of these folks you need to check your schedule first before you can commit. Those who are most comfortable leaning on you are the same people who enable you to stay deep in your disease to please.

But wait, you can't blame them. Flip that vanity mirror around and take a look at yourself. You've "yes'ed" your way right into this role. Starting today, you'll learn to politely decline your way into recovery!

Be kind and confidently hold your ground and remember that practice makes perfect. You're on the road to recovery!

Tips for Using TGR

- Practice saying the phrase (Thanks for thinking of me. Let me check my schedule and get back to you.) out loud, using your own words.

- There's no need to offer details or explain why you're too busy to say yes; people will rarely if ever ask why or challenge your response.

- You will feel an immediate sense of relief each time you use TGR.

- When you feel misplaced guilt, review your list of goals as a reminder of how valuable your time is in the pursuit of the life you've designed.

- In the rare instance that someone expresses disappointment in your reply, ask yourself if this person really wants the best for you or if the "disapproval" is self-serving.

Daily**PUSH**

1. Repeat this phrase, "Thanks for thinking of me! Let me check my schedule and I'll get back to you!"

2. Take a look at your inbox or text messages. Find as many opportunities as possible to reply with this phrase!

NOTES

_____

_____

_____

_____

_____

_____

_____

Consider the Consequence of Your Reply

Ever spent some time around teenagers? If so, you know there are certain phrases and replies that become habitual.

There was a period of about 3 weeks where my son Brock replied "Huh?" to everything. It didn't matter if it was a question or a statement. It made no difference if I was a foot from him with direct eye contact or a few feet away. His every reply was "Huh?" It mystified Bret and me. We wondered if we should take him for a hearing test. That's when my friend Barbie, who had raised two teens of her own, pointed out it was a common habit for teen boys, in exactly the same way our daughter, Cierra, can find a way to insert "like" six or seven times into just one sentence.

The phrases and replies we use are habits. I doubt that Brock would have picked up the same habit if we were raising him in Texas, where young adults habitually reply, "Ma'am?" or "Excuse me, ma'am?" Habit. Well, we didn't ship Brock off to Dallas, but we did offer some consequences if he didn't immediately drop the bad habit.

Weigh your own consequences. When I check my inbox each day, there are no fewer than 10 opportunities to say yes to someone I actually know and like: business associates, the team mom, customers, people I might feel I owe a favor, professional peers, etc. Recently, one such e-mail from a gal I used to teach with asked that I come and do an appearance at the grand opening for her new fitness studio, just 15 miles away. It sounded so simple. How could I not say yes? But her grand opening fell on a Saturday in a month when my schedule was beyond tight. I had scarcely enough time to sit and relax with my family. Though the opening was proposed as just an "hour" of my time, in reality I knew it would take 3 or 4 hours. To find the courage to use the right reply, I thought of my kids. I thought about spending time with Bret. What was more important during such a busy time, doing a favor for a fitness peer or having those extra hours to spend with family? What message would I be sending my family (even subliminally) if I had said yes to her? Considering the consequences of accepting her request gave me the confidence to use TGR.

When you're torn, when you can't decide on the right reply, look at your priorities. Tough decisions and the right reply are made simple when you have your priorities to guide you.

DAY 27
Cultivate
CONFIDENCE

Go Bold or Go Home!

I think we can all agree that confidence is one of the most attractive characteristics in another human being. I can't tell you how many times I've heard someone tell me, "I don't have the confidence to do a video." Or "I would love to follow my dreams, but I have really low self-esteem."

I'm not going to tell you to be more confident. That's silly. Instead, I'm going to give you action steps. Today I'm sharing with you the habits that build confidence. I'm going to give you the proven steps to boost your self-esteem and cultivate the confidence habit.

Confidence is not something you can buy or that you're born with. It's not something that you gain from having more money or more things or enjoying a certain lifestyle. All of us know some-one who is beautiful, thin, smart, and kind yet lacks confidence. I bet you also know someone who is overweight, not that attractive, but wildly successful and liked by all, and it's all because that person exudes confidence.

Confident people have more opportunities. They have greater success. They enjoy life. They have longer-lasting relationships. They give others confidence. If you want what they have, read on. You can have it!

Build Confidence One Action at a Time

So how does an adult build confidence? Are you ready? It's a one-letter word that begins with an *A!*

Action.

Yes, action builds confidence. Every time you set out to do something and you do it, whether you know it or not, you make a deposit into your confidence account. The more confident you are, the more confident people you'll draw into your life.

I want you to take note of how you're starting to feel about your own confidence level. Have you felt a general increase in your self-esteem as you work through this 30-day process?

Confidence comes from doing things that are scary, realizing that you survived and that everything is okay, and then doing it again. All while patting yourself on the back and saying, "Nice job!"

A critical step of using action to gain confidence happens when you recognize the action steps you've already taken. Give yourself credit for getting this far in the book! Congratulate yourself for any new habit or improved way of thinking that is starting to form.

You can never have too much confidence. You might disagree and ask, "Oh really? Because I know people who have so much confidence that they're arrogant SOBs." I'll bet if you peel away the layers of that onion, you're dealing with someone who's actually very insecure. Arrogance and confidence are not one and the same.

Confident individuals are comfortable to be around because they're happy in their own skin. They're good at being who they are. They don't feel the need to prove themselves or pee on trees to mark their territory. They don't worry about whether others like or don't like them. They're good with themselves.

Confidence is not something someone else can give or take away from you. One thing I've never allowed my kids to say is say is "so-and-so made me feel bad." No one can make you feel bad except you. Never give someone else the power to decide your confidence. You have to feel confident about yourself, and you do that not by the way you look, the things you own, the education you have, the money in your bank account.

You build confidence by doing. You have to believe that what you're doing is right. And if it's not right, you fix it.

The actions you have taken up to this point should give you a great sense of accomplishment. You're moving forward in a way that is consistent with your priorities. Every time you make a decision that is aligned with your priorities, feel the confidence that action creates.

Confidence Is Yours to Create

Confidence is not a trait that you're born with, that you can buy at the store, or that you can pretend to have. Confidence is *made*—and you're the only one who can make it.

Most psychiatrists and psychologists have

their own theories on self-confidence and security. I'm not a psychiatrist or psychologist. But I have spent the past 20 years studying what makes one person average and another person highly successful, and I've interviewed hundreds of individuals who describe themselves as once having had zero confidence and who now have the charismatic confidence that draws other people and amazing opportunities to them.

What does confidence look like? We sometimes picture a self-assured life of the party, someone who boldly walks to the center of the conversation, captures everyone's attention, and launches into a captivating story. We assume confident people are loud, gregarious, and entertaining. They love a crowd.

The truth is, confident people are easy to be around. They seem comfortable in their own skin. You don't feel like they're judging you.

Those with high self-esteem are often presented with the best opportunities. They're in the top of their industry. They're magnetic. They draw movers and shakers. They have incredible lives, and much of it is because of the positive energy they exude and attract.

Your confidence begins with your beliefs about yourself. Whatever you believe to be true about yourself becomes your reality. If you tell yourself that you're shy or you're insecure or you're uncomfortable around people you don't know, that is your reality.

In mulling over all of the interviews I have conducted on this topic, I noticed certain productive behavior patterns that I'm passing along to you. Here are the detailed action steps of those who developed the habits to build their confidence from the ground up.

Do Something Scary

Do something you fear. Make up your mind to feel the fear and just jump. The scarier, the better. For one individual, that was overcoming her fear of public speaking. For my friend Toni, a single mother of seven, it was overcoming the fear of going back to school.

Everything you do for the first time involves a degree of fear. Do you remember learning to ride a bike? You've been walking for only a few years when some adult decides you're going to learn to balance on an unstable moving metal device with wheels and steering and pavement to cushion your fall. Heck, when I was growing up, we didn't even have helmets. Now that's scary! But we did it and we survived and did it again and again and before long we had enough confidence to take it to the next level: "Look, Mom! No hands!"

The first time I did a live television appearance, as I stood off-set moments before my segment, I was sweating and shaking. The producer asked, "Are you scared?" I replied, "Nope, I'm excited!" Sure, I had butterflies, dry mouth, and uncontrollable shaking, but I knew this experience would make me stronger. I kept telling myself, "You're not nervous. You're excited. You're *excited!*" The side effects are virtually the same. When you're excited about doing something, how do you feel? Your heart races, your pulse quickens, and your body feels a little shaky. That's the way you feel when you're excited!

So from now on, don't tell yourself you're nervous or scared. Convince yourself that you're *excited*. And as soon as your feet hit the ground and you realize how petty your fears were, do it again and again and again, and you'll keep getting better. Whatever that fear is, conquer it. The scarier it is, the more confidence you will feel.

Seek Knowledge

Whether it's going back to school or really investigating the Bible or studying nutrition or learning a trade, when you gain knowledge, you gain confidence.

Having knowledge gives us confidence. Find something that you're passionate about and become an expert. Research all there is to know on the subject. Enroll in a class. Learn a new skill.

Live with Authenticity

Whenever you try to be somebody you're not, you automatically feel less secure. You just have to face it. Not everybody is going to like you. You can't be everyone's cup of tea. But when you are *you*, you make it easier for people to find you. We have limited time on this planet. You don't need 50 good friends. You don't even need 10 best friends. You just need a few people who genuinely want the best for you and push you to be authentically you. The rare but incredibly strong friendships you have are the ones that count. Stop trying to please everybody. You be you. Try it. I think you'll like it.

Run with the Stallions

How can you run like a stallion if you're busy hauling hay with the donkeys? If the people you're hanging with are negative Debbie downers, people who dislike themselves, you're taking on their negative belief systems, realize it or not.

Perhaps it's time to spend more time with the people who raise the bar. The folks in your life (and you have them if you're willing to look) who really are going places expect the most of themselves. You need a group of people who best represent the amazing person you're becoming.

Find a new group of people to hang out with. Wash yourself of negative thinkers and excuse makers. Read the books. Take the courses. Be dissatisfied with "good enough." Want more. Expect more. Improve yourself. Listen to self-improvement CDs and meet people who do the same. Listening to audio programs can change your thinking and motivate you to do what others will not dare push themselves to try.

Talk It Out

The last and most important action step for any of the individual suffering from fear, anxiety, or damaged self-esteem is to find a therapist. Tracking down the right professional is the key, and sometimes it takes visiting a few and doing a little homework in order to get the right fit. Lose the ego. You wouldn't walk around with a toothache for years; you'd find a professional to fix your pain. It's interesting to me that our emotions and past traumas can result in obesity, damaged relationships, years of depression, anxiety, and low self-esteem, yet so few people are willing to give therapy a try, or maybe another chance.

You don't want to "dump" your problems or divulge your personal demons to your friends, and to be honest, they are no more qualified to help you deal with your issues than they are to perform a root canal. Pain and trauma erode your self-esteem and damage your relationships. It is the ultimate act of selflessness to put your fears aside and find someone who is qualified to help.

Confidence is a habit created by boldly taking action. Today, make plans to do a few of the things (or even just one) you know you must, despite your fear.

You have an obligation to the people in your life to make this happen. If you want to do more for other people, you must believe in yourself—and that belief starts with you!

Daily**PUSH**

1. What are you secretly afraid to try but know that it would make you a more confident person?

2. Schedule your first attempt.

NOTES

_____

_____

_____

_____

_____

_____

_____

_____

DAY 28

Layers of
ACCOUNTABILITY

*Build a Wall of Resolve—
Brick by Brick*

Today we build a brick wall around your resolve. Accountability is what we'll call it, but I want you to think of it as both incentive and insurance.

Everyone knows establishing accountability helps us to stay the course, even when our former ways tempt us. If a little accountability is good, and more is better, than a mountain is what we'll create.

You're far more likely to adhere to your habits when you create a fortress of accountability around them. And the strongest form of accountability comes from outside ourselves.

Snag a Workout Buddy

Those who embark on a fitness journey with a friend, spouse, or family member have nearly double the success rate of someone who doesn't,

statistics show. A neighbor, your BFF, or even one of your Facebook friends who agrees to work out with you will help to ensure your adherence. Ask this person for a 6-month commitment, after which the two you can continue on or find another pushy partner!

This relationship goes both ways. Your partner must promise not to let you off the hook when you think you're too tired or too busy to exercise. You'll do the same for her or him.

Keep a Food Journal

This one is nonnegotiable. Believe me, I know the hardest part of counting calories is remembering

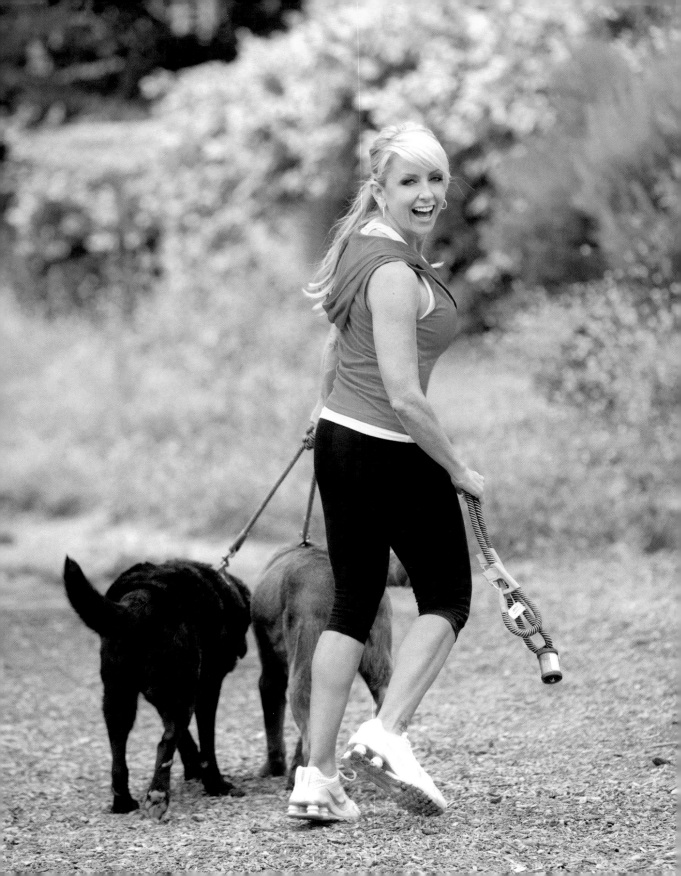

to do it. Balancing your checkbook isn't a whole lotta fun either, but both are necessary if you don't want to end up in big trouble.

Listen, if you're anything like me, you can barely remember where you parked, let alone every piece of food you eat. But you *must* know, and with relative accuracy. Why? Because just 100 calories more than you need each day can result in a 10-pound weight gain in just 1 year. Even if no one saw you eat those Hershey's Kisses or the crust from your kid's PB&J, the calories count and they add up fast. So buy yourself a cute portable notebook or download an app.

Honestly, keeping your journal on your phone with an app is really the easiest the way to go! A couple of the more popular ones on the iPhone are Calorie Tracker and Lose It! Since you have the Internet at your fingertips, you no longer have an excuse for not knowing how many calories any food item contains. The answer is only one little Google search away. Not to fear, Crackberry lovers! You have plenty of apps to choose from, too! And even more when you come to your senses and join our little iPhone cult.

Take a Picture of Yourself

You: Nooooooo!

Me: Yesssss!

No worries! Technology will make it painless! Just snap that photo yourself, in the privacy of your own bathroom, using your smartphone! No one but you will ever have to see it. Well, at least not until you're so blown away by your own results that you're pulling out your "before" photo to inspire others.

Recently I watched this amazing video titled *365 Days of Fitness*. In it, a man has taken a picture of himself, shirtless, postworkout, every day from day 1 to day 365 to document the slow and steady progression of his journey. He then assembled the photos in a manner to fly by in fast rotation. You literally feel like you're watching the story of the incredibly shrinking and shredding man!

So throw on a bathing suit, set up your camera, and snap some pics. Once a week, snap another pic wearing the same suit. This will allow you to see with certainty the amazing progress you're making!

Notice I said bathing suit. Do *not* wear your underwear. I'm not kidding. First, if I have to see one more sad-faced overweight person in a pair of skivvies, I'm gonna pinch someone's head off! Second, there will come a day when you will *want* to show the world how far you've come—trust me—and you will not want to share those photos if you're wearing your underwear.

You may not be happy with what you see today, but that too can be used to keep you motivated. Keep the photo on your phone where no one else will find it except you. Look at it when you're tempted to make poor food choices. Thinking about turning into the parking lot at Baskin-Robbins? What does today's photo think of that?

Make a Public Proclamation

When you share your goals with others, people genuinely want to see you succeed. When you make your goals a matter of public record (i.e., posting it on Facebook, announcing it at your family dinner, sharing your goals with co-workers, etc.), you enlist others in your hopes. The integrity of your word and your proclamation shore up your intentions and motivate you to make it happen.

Draw Up an Accountability Contract

Any successful transformation requires you to be fully committed to changing your lifestyle. By formally agreeing to a contract, you confirm your commitment to your goals. In the business world, it is not uncommon for penalties to apply when the terms of the contract are not met. It's one thing to sign an accountability contract, quite another to have serious consequences for not meeting the terms.

Accountability contracts can include just about any area. For example, you can incentivize your weight maintenance by signing a friendly contract to pay your workout partner $100 for every pound you gain over your target weight. That's motivation! Accountability contracts can be used to remind you to go to bed with your spouse, wake early, and exercise or reach a business objective. Where do you find one? Google it!

Join an Online Support Group

Being part of an online community (some charge; some are free) will keep you accountable,

and you can check in when your schedule permits. These sites often offer live chat forums, videos, recipes, experts, and motivation. And the communities on some of these sites are so powerful that their success stories will blow your mind. If you're looking for inspiration, you'll find it on these forums!

Many sites also provide online weight-loss support and tools such as BMR calculators, contests, message boards, and more to help you through your journey, which is an awfully strong layer of accountability. I particularly love the user-generated weight-loss support forums. You can choose between professional weight-loss support or simply share ideas, motivation, and support with others just like you!

- http://dailyburn.com
- www.onlinefitnesslog.com
- www.sparkpeople.com
- www.myyogaonline.com
- www.beachbody.com
- www.3fatchicks.com
- www.30daypush.com

Join a Group Fitness Class

There are many advantages to group exercise and group fitness classes. One major benefit is the motivation you'll gain from working out with others. Statistics show the average person works with greater intensity and for longer periods of time when he or she exercises with others. The group that you work out with often forms a

Pay It Forward

Have you ever noticed when you're watching one of the recovery addiction programs that the counselors tend to be recovering addicts themselves? Weight-loss coaches are often successfully healthy people who are now teaching others how to master their own weight. Placing yourself in the role of teacher, mentor, or coach places a great deal of responsibility on your shoulders. It forces you to be accountable. Why do you think I teach workout classes every day of the week?

family and a system of support. You'll forge friendships and networking opportunities that will last a lifetime.

Miss a workout and you're likely to be greeted with "Hey, where were you yesterday?" The unspoken expectation that you'll be there is powerful! The variety and social nature of group classes will keep things interesting. Even as a fitness professional, I find that the classes that I teach keep me inspired and in check.

Tweet Your Progress

There are countless ways to use the watchful eyes of your friends in social media to keep you accountable. Ask your virtual friends for their assistance in keeping your eyes on the prize. Consider a daily tweet with your weight, take a picture of yourself postworkout, create a Facebook album with your progress photos.

Here's what happens when you share your journey in social media: People cheer, support, and find inspiration from you. When you receive a Facebook inbox from someone so profoundly touched by your photos or your story, it

becomes bigger than you. Nothing creates accountability and motivation like knowing someone, even a virtual friend, is inspired by your journey.

Check Out Online Coaching

I'm a huge fan of coaching! Even though I've been public speaking for more than 15 years, I use a speaking coach. Even after two of my infomercials reached number one, I hired an on-camera coach to learn to better connect on screen. A good coach will push you to reach your potential, help you make informed decisions about your career, business, or financial goals. The right coach becomes your sounding board and your voice of reason. A coach will keep you accountable and will continually raise the bar. You will benefit from their experience, expertise, and networking opportunities. The best part of working with a coach is what I call the "winning record" incentive. That is to say that coaches, and especially the

(continues on page 198)

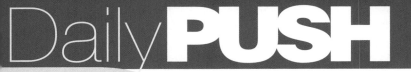

Join or Create a Mastermind!

What's a mastermind? It's a group of people who commit to push each other. They may or may not have similar goals, but what they share in common is their commitment to push each other. Think of it as a support group where excuses won't fly! *Mastermind* is a term originally coined by Napoleon Hill in his timeless classic *Think and Grow Rich* in which he encouraged people to come together to create synergistic energy and momentum toward their goals.

I've been running masterminds for years and can tell you it is one of the most rewarding and valuable investments of my time. Even though I consider myself a highly motivated, goal-oriented individual, the accountability of a small group that meets on a regular schedule to evaluate each other's progress is extremely inspiring.

When it comes to "goal getting," a group of motivated individuals meeting once a week, maybe once a month to push each other, offer feedback, support, and accountability is unbelievably effective. In a mastermind or whatever *you* want to call your group of movers and shakers, you'll be accountable to people who, like you, want to be pushed to reach their goals professionally as well as personally.

I call my own weekly group the Three Percenters (referring to the small percentage of people who actually follow a system of written goal mastery). I selected each person first of all because I really like each of them, they're all serious about getting serious, and most important, they're each the type of individual who wants to help others but wouldn't be afraid to voice an opinion if a fellow member wasn't living up to his or her potential! Each of us is from a different perspective. With members ranging from experienced business owners to a stay-at-home mom looking to turn her hobby into an enterprise, a mastermind will expose you to unique opinions and the experience of those from another industry or life perspective.

The Three Percenters meet once a week for 2 hours over 6 months. The idea is to have members push each other to achieve their goals, keep their word from the previous week, and network to help each other's businesses grow!

The new strategies and mutual excitement you feel as members of your group peck away at their goals will create momentum; forming or joining a mastermind skyrockets the speed of your success. When you commit to other successful people, you are more likely to follow through than if you just commit to yourself.

To find a mastermind group in your area, log on to Google and type "join mastermind [name of your city]." You might even want to start your own group. If you do, limit meetings to five or six people. Include members who are up and coming or well-established movers and shakers. Invite people with varying levels of success to make it fun for those with well-established success to mentor newbies. The Web site www.lifehack.org is a great place for ideas on selecting and running your own mastermind.

NOTES

_____

_____

_____

_____

_____

_____

_____

_____

_____

_____

_____

_____

_____

most successful coaches, have a vested interest in maintaining their winning streak. They want you to succeed! Talk to any people who have risen to the top of their profession, and you will find a great coach helped them to reach their potential.

If you're thinking of hiring a life coach, business coach, or fitness coach, a great solution is online coaching done via phone, e-mail, Skype, and Ustream. Many people enjoy the anonymity and (relative) affordability of using an online coach.

Coaching services can range from free to $150 per hour. Before you hire a coach, do your research. Ask for recommendations, and never commit to advance payment until you feel you've had enough time to determine if your coach has the qualities you need.

Daily**PUSH**

1. List each one of these layers of accountability on your to-do list.

2. Move two of these items to your Today list and the remaining to "This Month."

NOTES

_____

_____

_____

_____

_____

_____

_____

_____

Find a Therapist

You might wonder why I would list a therapist as a source of accountability. For starters, if you have struggled with food addiction, body issues, fear of success, or self-doubt, these issues may be the result of early traumas in your life. A therapist will not only help you to solve the issues that are causing you to turn to food but also may help you to deal permanently with a matter that otherwise might sabotage your success.

Whatever you want to label it, "letting yourself go," "getting fat," or "obese," your physical condition probably has very little to do with just "lacking willpower." Most experts agree that obesity often leads to or results from an addiction, an addiction to food. For the food addict, cravings are as powerful and life altering as those an alcoholic or drug addict experiences. Joining a support group or reorganizing your pantry is like putting a bandage on a hemorrhaging wound. Not going to cut it. If you have *demons,* unresolved issues that continue like a beach ball to surface despite your best efforts to push them below the surface, I urge you to find a qualified individual to help you. While society doesn't always understand the issues, food addiction experts know the inner struggles that compulsive overeaters and those who suffer from eating disorders face.

Therapy is like dental care. Don't expect to "fix it," brush your hands together, and walk away forever. You'll need a checkup from time to time. A great therapist will keep you accountable.

Spirituality and Religion

Having a spiritual connection or religious affiliation offers a wonderful source of support. Spirituality can offer a sense of hope and purpose in our life and help us find greater strength and resilience. You can also connect with a community of others who have similar beliefs. Do some research; your church probably offers support and small groups for those looking for accountability on their weight-loss journey. Why stop there? There's more to this journey than health and fitness. If your faith provides you with the strength to do anything, why not find a faith-based group that aligns with your Push goal?

EMERGENCY 911!

In the Event of a Slip, Break Open This Chapter

> "When you come to the end of your rope,
> tie a knot and hang on."
>
> —Franklin D. Roosevelt

I'm so glad you're reading this today. Why? Because I have to tell you how amazing you are! Seriously.

I don't know if you know this or not, but very few people make it to Day 29 on their first go at this. Why? A variety of reasons, the greatest of which is that they don't believe they deserve the life of their design. They don't believe that spending 5 or 10 minutes a day is worthwhile to achieve whatever it is they want to have happen in the next 12 months. But you get it, and I love you for that. You are in an elite group of people who follow through and do not quit!

If you slip, don't be fazed. Readjust your gaze on your destination and continue forward. Keep moving. You are not a quitter. You can do anything. Success is your only option. Yes, even successful people make mistakes. They have bad days. They slip up. But on the flip side, they persist and never give up. You're kicking some serious tail right now, so don't get flustered.

The greater your effort, the greater your reward. You made a promise to yourself and others that this time would be different. The easiest way to honor your promise to yourself and your important people is simply to resolve to never, ever quit. This is your destiny, and you're so much closer than you think.

Have a Mantra

When I ran cross-country in high school, I remember our coach running up to those of us straggling along in the back. Repeatedly he'd yell, "You're not tired! You're not tired!" I was certainly not a cross-country star, but his mantra stuck with me. I've been repeating those words to myself for years.

One day, during the final minutes of filming a 60-minute Turbo Jam video, the words I repeat in my head to keep myself going somehow came out of my mouth: "You are not tired!" I yelled into the lens of the camera. Didn't even think about it at the time, but I later learned from thousands of fans that the phrase I borrowed from my mild-mannered high school cross-country coach proved just as motivating to them as it was to me.

Create your own mantra. Think of something that will keep you going when you want to quit.

"Just keep swimming, just keep swimming, just keep swimming, swimming, swimming," my kids have borrowed from *Finding Nemo*.

And lest we not forget *The Little Engine That Could*, "I think I can, I think I can . . ."

When I find myself discouraged by setbacks, I repeat to myself, "I may not have their good fortune, but in the end I will prevail through persistence." Or "I'm very close. I'm very close." Whatever works for you will do just that. Work hard. Dig deep. I will do this!

You have made it through the tough stuff.

Now, I couldn't tell you before you started this challenge that the first 10 days were going to be gnarly—that could have been kinda daunting and you might not have believed me when I told you how totally worth it everything would be. But you did! You made it through! You made it through the hardest part—the part where, quite honestly, we weed out the people who are quitters.

And you are still with it. You are in this to win it. And now, you can start to feel that momentum, right? Don't you feel you are already moving in a different direction? Like the momentum starts to build behind you to the point where you don't even have to keep running. It's as if it's pushing you toward the things you want to happen this year. It's not in your mind. This is really happening.

Success is not a place at which one arrives but rather the spirit with which one undertakes and continues the journey.
—Author unknown

Decide Not to Slide

Don't let a slip turn into a slide. This isn't a diet. This isn't a short-term exercise in goal setting. This is a way of life. Success is formed of the habits you've developed and the knowledge you have gained. There are going to be days where you don't get your exercise in. Or you've eaten something that you know you probably shouldn't have. Don't sweat it.

The dieter's mentality is that "if I've had one or two or three cookies, I've blown it. Might as well eat the whole box." And that turns into "Well, I've blown it today. I might as well spend the rest of my week punishing myself by eating bad food, and I'll start my diet next week." That's called a slide. This is a way of life. Believe it or not, you're human. You're gonna miss the occasional workout. You're going to enjoy the occasional treat. You can do those things in moderation.

Slips Happen, So What?

Starting now, you'll recognize that when you start to slip off your bike, instead of falling, you right yourself and focus straight ahead.

There are times when you mess up in life. Have you ever lost your temper with someone you love? (Naw, nobody does that. Ever.) But here on Earth, when that happens, you snap yourself out of it. You're motivated to immediately stop your bad behavior because you know you may have hurt someone you love. You check yourself, apologize, and get yourself back in line.

Funny how we don't always do that when the behavior is hurtful to ourselves. That must change. When your "slip" happens, realize that you are hurting yourself and stop it in its tracks. When you have a not-so-healthy dinner, start the next day with a superhealthy breakfast. When you realize you've gone 2 days without checking or creating a daily to-do list, don't let it slide—get back into the habit the very next day!

Everything counts. You're doing your best! Slip up, but forge ahead. Don't let a slip turn into a slide. You're so close!

Daily PUSH

1. Create your own mantra to inspire you when things get tough.

2. Pat yourself on the back! You are in an elite group of successful people!

NOTES

_____

_____

_____

_____

_____

_____

BUBBLE-WRAP
Your Success

Respect It, Protect It, Go Get It!

Today is Review Day. It's also an opportunity to remind yourself of how far you've come and the amazing opportunities that lie before you, along with learning some suggestions on how to "bubble-wrap" your progress!

As you embark on your 30th day, are you basking in the glow of all you've learned? Are you implementing your new tools? If so, how hard are you rockin' 'em? If not, that's okay. Embrace your open mind. Let all of the previous 29 days start to marinate; think about them, sleep on it, then reread and maybe take some notes.

Now that you have actually gone through the process, you're seeing how every piece affects the next and how much control you really do have over your destiny. You look at everyday life just a little differently. You have a sense of calm and

confidence and an inner energy all at once.

You're responding differently to people. You're kinder and more patient. You've begun to like yourself and understand how important it was to get your priorities straight before you tackled another diet! People have noticed a change. (Shoot! You've only just begun!) How you set goals and tackle your daily assignments will never be the same. You're on your way, kid!

Go ahead! You're experienced enough now. Go back and reread some stuff. I promise you, you'll pick up some details that you missed the

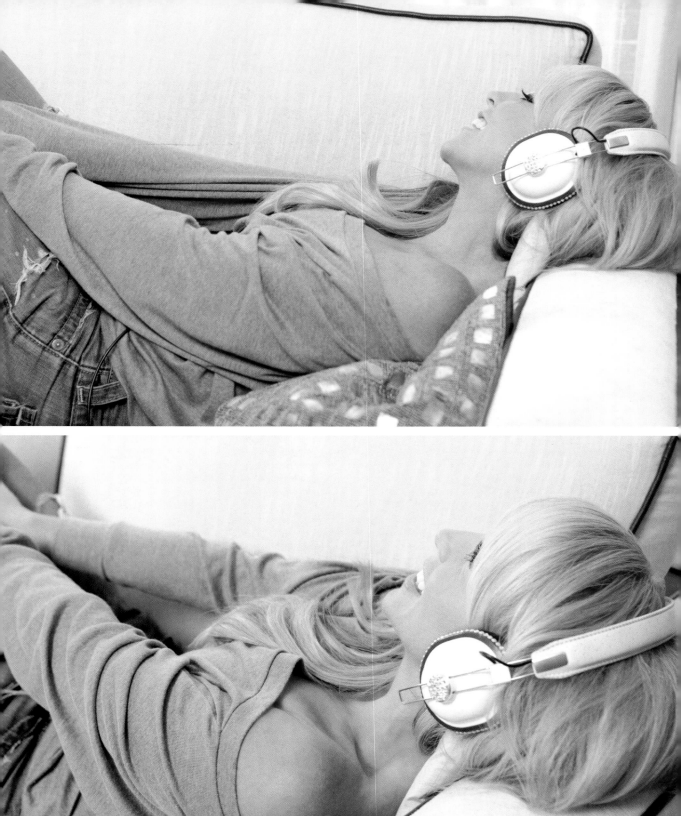

first time. That's the best way to learn: Let the message sink in a little bit, live it, experience it, go back and review it, and then rewrite your notes.

These are probably the most important 30 days of your year. You learned that you have the skills to do anything. While some of the information is stuff you already knew or have done before, you simply needed that reminder, a little something that pulled it all together and—of course—the Push. So today, what I want to do is go through a quick review of what we've covered up to this point.

Priorities

We started with your *priorities*, the guiding principles of your life. They're not goals. They are the way you intend to live your life. Your priorities are things that you neither would nor could sacrifice. So when you listed your order of priorities, that first thing at the tippy top of your list (that one thing that you would not sacrifice no matter what) was the most important thing in your whole entire world. You then arranged the rest of your list in order of importance to yourself.

Voilà! Your guiding principles. Your priorities are what you used, and will continue to use, as a gauge to decide if your goals are consistent with such.

Goals

The *goals* that you set for yourself are measurable. They're actions that you must take to reach something in particular, something that you can quantify. To reach a certain dollar amount or a certain number of sales with your business, to spend x number of days on vacation next year, to pay off x number of dollars in your mortgage or buy a car without having to finance it—those are measurable goals.

Now, some of your goals are personal, some are professional, perhaps some are spiritual. Ultimately, all of them came from your desire to become a better person or to be more able to provide for your family. Once you created your list of goals, you looked at each one and then you looked at your priority list to see if said goals were aligned with your priorities.

Push Goal

Once you aligned your goals with your priorities, you picked the one or two goals that would make all (or at least most) of your other goals possible. Whatever your goals are, there's one on that list (maybe even two) that makes succeeding at all the others more likely. That's your Push goal.

Let's say that the most important goal on your list is to spend more time with your family. That's not your Push goal. A Push goal is one that, once obtained, makes it *possible* for you to spend more time with your family. Or reduce your stress. Or lose 100 pounds.

Remember, your Push goal should not be a skill. A skill is something you need to learn and acquire to help you *reach* your Push goal.

Your To-Do List

Then you developed a taste for action and started creating a to-do list at the same time and at the same place every day, and you kept it with you everywhere 24/7. And on your to-do list are two or three items that move you closer to your Push goal. You now notice these items every time you add something to your list or simply as you're checking your list throughout the day.

Yes, when you run into someone who says, "Hey, don't forget that meeting on Wednesday," as you're adding that meeting to your to-do list, you'll see your Push goal. Remember, each time you look at your to-do list, regardless of whether you're adding something or taking something off, one of the first things you see is your Push goal. And that's intentional, so that what you're thinking about the most becomes your reality.

Hopefully, you're now using digital technology to help you program your mind to think about the thing that is most important. And by most important, I mean your Push goal—again, the goal that makes most of the other things on your goal list possible.

Progress, Not Perfection

We've also realized that this journey you're on is a process. As I've shared with you, after I researched many of my own goals, I realized that the reality of some of them wasn't consistent with my priorities. So then it's time to shift.

Don't fight it. Don't be stubborn. Just say, "Hey, this doesn't work. So before I invest any more time, let me set up a new Push goal that's consistent with my priorities and values."

And in doing so, you feel harmony. Because it's not the money and it's not things and it's not even losing all the weight and having the perfect body-fat ratio that will bring you happiness. Happiness comes by creating balance, by creating the life that you designed, by having that control, and isn't it exciting? Isn't it cool to see this happening, like how much control you actually have?

The Importance of Action

You hear lots about the laws of attraction, but typically people think that means, "If I think about it, it will come to me." That's not true—*action* brings and attracts those things to you. And the first action step is putting it down on paper, in good ol' black and white, and then carrying it with you all the time on your phone or on your notebook so that you're thinking about it all the time. This is a process; each step has been critical in creating this undeniable success.

Your Soul-Mate Workout and Your Numbers

You have found your soul mate, and I'm hoping you are spending almost every day together. When you team your soul mate with the numbers you've figured out, you are *crushing* this formerly mysterious weight-loss thing! You are doing this. Organizing everything makes this so much easier, from your day to your newly rearranged fridge. It's all coming together.

Your Promises

You have also made promises to those who care about your well-being perhaps even more than do you. They are your cheerleaders, and you want to make them, and yourself, proud. We're all one big team who by establishing balance independently can function even more smoothly as a group. When we are balanced and happy, it's that much easier to endure that which is not within our control.

You can't be stopped. Because you realize you can't do everything, you can do anything! Your habits are among the elite. So few people take the time to learn this stuff. You are in a special class of people. Walk tall, but never be too proud to share!

You have the steps—there's no link missing. Embrace your ever-growing confidence and the knowledge that all things are possible when you practice your best habits. It is happening, and you have everything you need to know.

Today's Hug

No push today. Just a big bear hug! You no longer need pushing from me. You've got all the momentum you need to make this happen. I really wish I could give you a tight squeeze and let you know how much it means to me that you did the work, gave me your trust, believed in yourself, and made it 30 days!

Along with the hug, let me leave you with a few reminders. If you're reading this in digital form, copy, paste, print, and post on your wall. If you're reading an old-fashioned, real-pages-that-turn kinda book, then cut this box out and post it in the room where you spend the most time.

Success Reminders

1. Live to be better! You know you've figured out success when you realize there's always room for improvement. That's the journey. Strive for more.

2. Have regularly scheduled checkups every 3 months. Place a reminder on your phone to repeat the process every 3 months. You will pick up this book and do a quick skim. Even though you're not going anywhere but up from here, it never hurts to make sure you keep yourself in check!

3. Read, act, repeat. Repetition creates long-term memory grooves in your brain. To really make this stuff stick, do it again, then share it with other people—but make sure they buy their own book! You need this one!

4. Get a sponsor! Just as addicts need someone to help guide them as they change their ways, it's important for you to have a sponsor. Ask a key person to be the sponsor who has permission to set you straight should you fall off track.

5. Never give up! No matter what life throws at you—and it will, about every 2 months—never quit!

PART 2

3 CIRCUITS, ONE BANGIN' BODY!

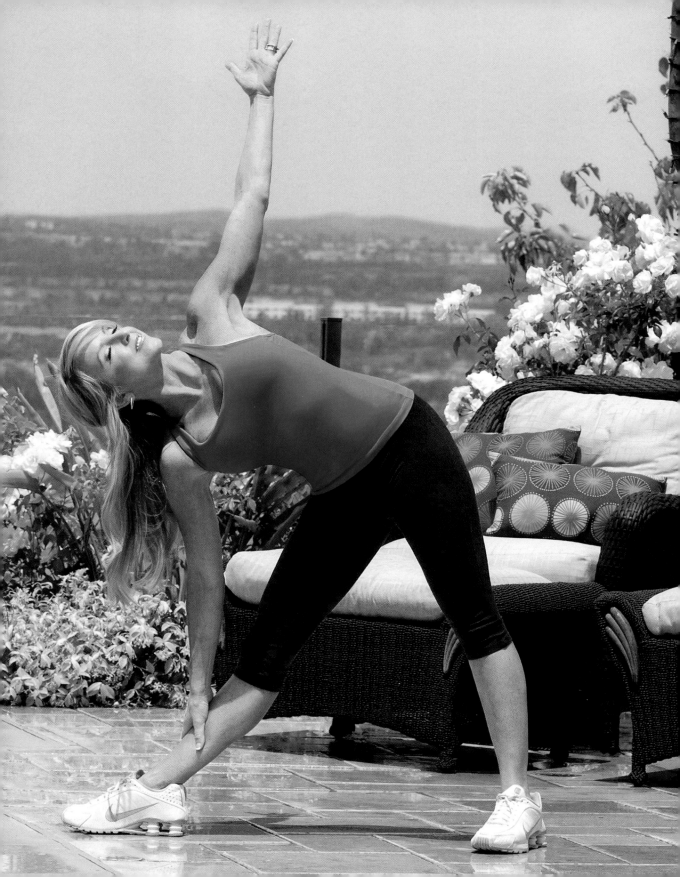

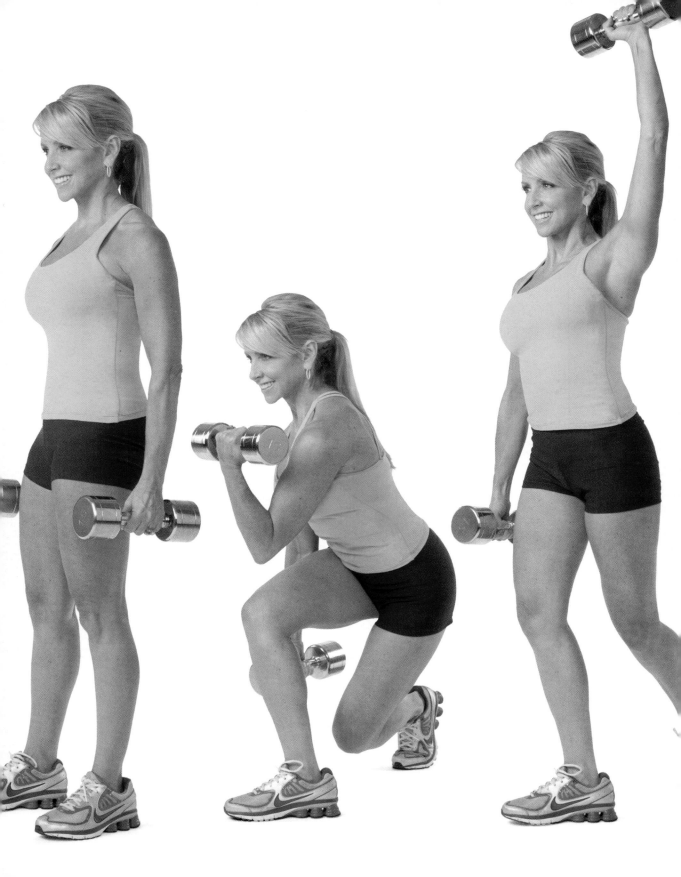

Before You Start

My love for strength training grew from my personal journey. When I began strength training in a way that was scientifically proven to provide the most effective results for fat loss, I knew that anyone could get results. I was compelled to embark on a mission to change people's minds about strength training, especially the physically inactive and women.

As I approached 40, I started noticing that my body was not quite responding to my "standard cardio" routine. It's not like there was anything drastically wrong, but I suddenly felt like my metabolism was slowing. I knew that I could look and feel better.

So I started doing a whole lot of research about body fat, our metabolism, and strength-training methods—not just by talking to other personal trainers but by actually hitting the books. I looked over the latest scientific studies and research, trying to figure out what the best methodology was for creating and keeping a long, lean, sculpted physique and really revving up the fat-burning machine.

Well, the main principle that kept recurring in all of my research was that building muscle tissue reduces body fat.

I put my money where my mouth was and assembled a test group of approximately 70 men and women of all shapes, sizes, and ages with a common commitment to change. These peeps committed to 3 days of strength training, 5 days of cardio workouts, and, of course, eating a healthy diet.

The results were nothing short of astonishing. Regardless of whether they were short, tall, old, or young, every single individual dramatically transformed their body composition. The group averaged a 50 percent loss of body fat, and their BMR (remember, that's basal metabolic rate) increased by *as much as 70 percent!*

Though any strength training is beneficial, slow, controlled reps working to create momentary failure in less than 12 reps is one of the best ways to improve muscular strength and therefore reduce body fat. However, if muscular endurance is your objective because, say, your goal is to improve your marathon time, you would use lighter weights, increased reps, and longer workout sessions.

In this section, I'm sharing with you some of the most effective strength-training exercises that the folks in this group used to transform their bodies. Those exercises can be used to customize your own bangin' body circuit program.

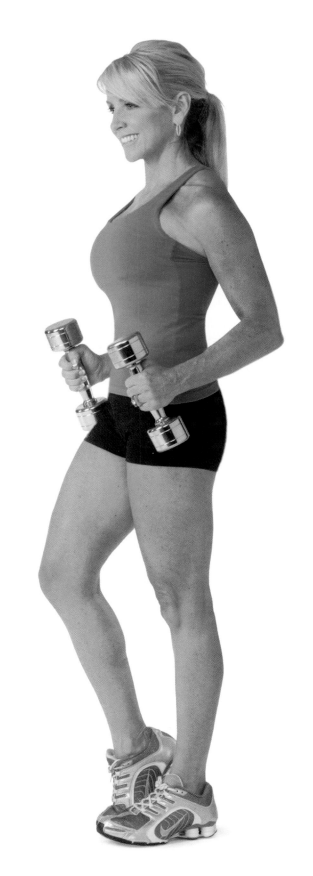

Fail to Win

For many of you, "failure" has a negative connotation, but failure during strength training is crucial for fast results. What is "failure" in weight training? Very simply, it means that your brain is telling your body to lift the weight, but your muscle is "done." This is validation that you have worked a muscle group with ultimate effectiveness. Optimal strength training for muscle development (which reduces body fat) should aim to fail between your 10th and 12th repetition.

Selecting Weights

Again, I'm going to assume here that you, like most people, are not training for an endurance event but training in a way that saves you time and reduces body fat. If that's the case, read on:

When you select a weight for a particular exercise, select one that is heavy enough to ensure that you *will* fail on your 10th, 11th, or 12th rep. If you have misjudged and picked up a weight that is too light, make note and go heavier next time.

Oh man, I can just hear some of you objecting to this concept, certain that you're going to "bulk up." But let me interject: No matter how heavy you lift, the process of building muscle takes time. You will not wake up tomorrow, look in the mirror, and say, "Oh no! My muscles are huge!" It doesn't work that way. Muscle growth is a process.

Trust me when I say this has worked for thousands of people, real people just like you. Apply the following components to your strength training and your results will far exceed your expectations:

- *Periodization*—Changes it up every 30 days.
- *Heavier weights*—Accelerates results with shorter workouts.
- *Slow, controlled movement*—Minimizes injury, promotes fiber recruitment.
- *Failure*—The quicker you reach muscle failure, the faster you get results.
- *Weight training is sexy*—Women get smaller, men get ripped!

Your Bangin' Body Workout Schedule

For someone as smart, productive, and motivated as you are, 30 minutes of daily exercise is simply nonnegotiable. If you were interested in having a baseline of health, we would start there.

You have concrete goals that go beyond just "being healthy." If you want to be in the best shape of your life, you have to put in the work to deserve it! So here goes (and trust me, this looks far worse on paper than it really is) . . .

Optimally, you're working to get to a point where every day you're doing something that makes you feel great. A week should look something like this:

3 **strength circuits** of approximately 30 minutes each (90 minutes total)

3 **intense,** short-duration cardiovascular workouts (25 to 40 minutes)

2 **moderate-intensity,** long-duration cardiovascular workouts (45 to 90 minutes)

1 **moderate- to low-intensity** cardiovascular activity for 30 minutes or more

1 or 2 flexibility workouts, postcardiovascular exercise (20 minutes minimum)

Ideally, you'll do your flexibility workout immediately after a cardiovascular workout. This will save you time, as you're already sweaty, warm, and ready to improve your flexibility.

How long should your workouts be? Just start. If you can't do 30 minutes of intense exercise, do 30 minutes of moderate exercise, but for the love of God, please stop treating yourself like anything other than an athlete.

You've seen the weight-loss competition shows. Wouldn't you love to have their results? Well, you can if you follow their general guiding philosophy, which is to treat contestants not like fat people but like the athletes they will become.

Treat yourself like a fat person with aches and pains and a suitcase full of excuses, and good luck—you'll stay exactly where you are. Train like an athlete and, though you may not look like one now, you will become one.

Start where you can and work your way up to the Bangin' Body Formula. If you can do 10 minutes three times a day to begin, do it! But each day, you'll add a minute until you reach 30, then 60. Gradually increase the duration and intensity of your workouts, then increase the number of days until you are active 7 days a week.

These 3 circuit workouts will seriously kick your butt, but you're done in 20 to 30 minutes, once you know what you're doing! Get your session out of the way first thing in the a.m. or right after your cardio! Typically, you won't get too sweaty, making it easier to get back to work or on with your day. A bangin' body mandates that

you become a stickler for good form, so go slow. Yes, going slower is definitely tougher, but it's also safer. Here's the crazy part about going slow . . . your muscles actually fatigue faster! By reaching muscle fatigue sooner, you'll be able to shorten your workouts.

I've designed your bangin' body circuits to hit all of your major muscle groups in just three workouts! Since you'll be strength training 3 days a week—let's say Monday, Wednesday, and Friday—you'll see that each circuit has been designed to target and define a different set of muscles. However, what all 3 circuits have in common is what I call "multitasking muscle work":

1. You'll work upper body and lower body at the same time for maximum calorie burn as well as a moderate cardio effect.

2. Exercises have been designed to challenge your core, while targeting an upper-body muscle group and keeping the lower body loaded.

3. You'll get to "pick any pushup." (Yup! Aren't you lucky? *You're welcome!*)

I've selected the exercises that will give you the best results in the least amount of time with nothing more than your body weight and a set of dumbbells or exercise tubing.

Each circuit begins with a 5-Minute Warmup (pages 225–228). Don't skip your warmup! The warmup will help you get the most out of your strength training and stay injury free. Each circuit consists of approximately 6 exercises. For each exercise, you'll do 12 to 15 reps, unless indicated otherwise. In all circuits, you'll do two exercises, then a set of pushups (make it your goal to work up to 12 pushups per set).

Failure Is the Key to Lean

Back to the number of reps you'll do per exercise . . . this is important. The number of reps you plan to do determines how much weight you should select. Keep in mind that muscle "failure" is your goal. Your muscles can't count; instead, they respond to "overload." In other words, your goal is to select enough resistance (i.e., a heavy enough weight) to create momentary muscle fatigue somewhere between 11 and 15 reps. To get maximum benefit from these circuits, select a weight that is challenging for you.

As a point of reference, I use from 12- to 20-pound dumbbells for the exercises in these circuits, but you'll need to find the right weights for your level of fitness . . . somewhere between Barbie Doll and No Chance! You want to select a weight heavy enough so that you can just *barely* do the 12th rep! Momentary muscle fatigue–induced failure should occur between the 10th and 12th rep. If you feel as though you could do a few more reps after 12, consider using a heavier weight next time.

Are these circuits tough? Oh yeah, but they're quick! Your arms will shake, and you may experience momentary muscle fatigue failure. But that's good—that's the *goal*! Still, if you want or need an easier workout, feel free to stretch the 20 minutes into an hour until you get stronger. Once that happens, I'm betting that you'll love that you can maintain your bangin' bod in an hour a week!

Working the Circuit

Each circuit will take you about 20 minutes to complete once you get familiar with each exercise. Allow for about double that the first couple of times you go through each circuit, as you'll probably want to refer to the instructions and photos, especially if you're new to this whole fitness thing. (Have an extra 5 minutes? Use that time to stretch postworkout to minimize soreness and maximize strength!)

Take the time you need to work with good form. But *do* try to complete the circuits without resting between exercises. And keep the following tips in mind—they'll help you get the most from your workout.

GO SLOW Perform each exercise as if you're moving underwater in slow motion. This eliminates the assistance of momentum that makes most workouts less effective. Slow, slow, slow is the way to go!

MAKE TRANSITIONS QUICK Even though you'll move with slow, controlled, and contracted muscles during each exercise, do the transition from one exercise to the next as quickly as possible. This will help you maintain a mild cardiovascular effect and burn more fat and calories.

NO BARBIE DOLL WEIGHTS This is so important, I needed to say it twice. To get lean, you gotta *Go heavy or go home!* I'm a little bossy about this because I've seen the science and I know how much faster you'll see results—just trust me on this one!

(continued on page 225)

PUSHUP GrabBag

Pushups Rock!

As you move through the circuits, you'll see that there are lots of pushups. I mean A LOT. You might be wondering why I've placed so much emphasis on the good old-fashioned pushup. Quite simply: They're one of the most effective ways to get a total upper-body workout and sculpt your core.

That said, I used to hate pushups. Even in my own classes, most of my students can do more pushups on their toes than yours truly. But even when I modify and go to my knees, the results I get in my upper body and abs are all the incentive I need to work at it. You *will* get stronger, your body *will* get leaner, and pushups will be your friend.

You might also be wondering why you have to do classic pushups when you could use an exercise machine or free weights—say, the bench press—to work the same muscle groups. My answer: because you won't get the same effect. The muscle that receives the most workout from a pushup are the pectoral muscles in

your chest (aka "pecs"), and the same is true for bench pressing. But pushups work your *whole body*. From head to toe, your body kicks into overdrive to support itself and maintain a stiff and straight posture—a task you don't have to do lying on your back to bench press.

Does this mean the more weight you have to lose, the harder pushups will be? Of course! But that's okay. If when I said, "Drop and give me 20," you smiled, obliged, and threw in a clap between each rep, I'd have to tell you to find a way to make what I've given you much harder. Remember, the harder your workout, the faster you'll see results.

While you do use your arm, pec, and shoulder muscles when you do pushups, your core does the real work. Your core is critical to creating a well-balanced body and to gaining the strength you need to perform all exercises with greater efficiency. Plus, when you have a strong core and defined upper body, you'll stand taller, improve your posture, boost your energy, and generally look thinner than someone of the

Tricep Pushup

1. Lie face down on your mat with your hands slightly wider than shoulder-width apart and under your chest. Keep your fingers straight and your legs straight and slightly apart with your toes supporting your feet. Your weight should be on your hands and toes.

2. Keep your body as straight as possible, with your eyes focused straight down and your neck in a neutral position.

3. Lower your chest toward the floor while keeping your arms close to your sides. Your elbows should be pointing straight back.

4. Squeeze your glutes and brace your abdominals throughout the pushup. Do not allow your lower back to sag or your hips to pike upward during the downward phase.

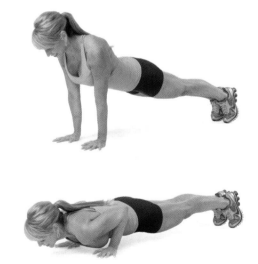

same weight with poor posture and a weak core. A strong core can banish back pain and make all your workouts safer and easier.

To get these benefits, you must maintain proper form: flat back, hands positioned under your shoulders. Different hand positions put different loads on your joints and muscles, but every one of us is put together a little differently. The way you need to place your hands to feel strongest might be slightly different than the way I need to keep my hands, so experiment with hand positions (as long as your hands are positioned under your shoulders).

However, it's vital to keep your back flat. It's challenging to do this, and it forces your abs to work their hardest. But making that effort will give you the greatest results. Poor posture all but undoes the work you're going through, so make sure to do it right!

Modified pushups, which you do on your knees, are virtually identical to normal pushups except that the muscles are worked at a lesser intensity or overload. It's important to maintain proper form in the modified position, too. Rest your weight slightly above your knees (not directly on your kneecaps), keep your back flat, and contract your abs.

If you're new to exercising, start with modified pushups and limit your range of motion. In due time, you'll be able to take your chest to the floor. Your goal, however, is to push yourself to go a little lower each time you go through these circuits. Your next step would be to start each set with the first rep on your toes, then move to your knees. Before long, you'll be doing the whole set on your toes with exceptional form. No matter how frustrating it is at first, every rep is changing your body! Pushups are tough. They're supposed to be. But you're tougher!

Here they are! As you move through the circuits, you can return to this "Pushups Rock!" sidebar and make your selections. It doesn't matter which you choose as long as you do them. As you find yourself getting more proficient, mix it up. If something feels difficult, that's a good indication that you're getting a solid workout.

Modified Tricep Pushup

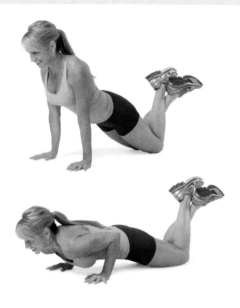

1. Get on your hands and knees, with your hands shoulder-width apart. Cross your feet at the ankles, creating a straight line from the top of your head to your knees.

2. Keep your body as straight as possible, with your eyes focused straight down and your neck in a neutral position.

3. Lower your chest toward the floor while keeping your arms close to your sides. Your elbows should be pointing straight back.

4. Squeeze your glutes and brace your abdominals throughout the pushup. Do not allow your lower back to sag or your hips to pike upward during the downward phase.

Traditional Pushup

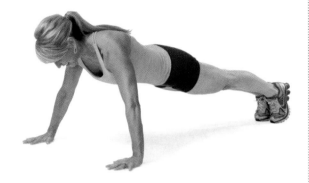

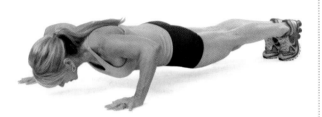

1. Lie face down on your mat with your hands slightly wider than shoulder-width apart and under your chest. Keep your fingers straight and your legs straight and slightly apart with your toes supporting your feet. Your weight should be on your hands and toes.

2. Keep your body as straight as possible, with your eyes focused straight down and your neck in a neutral position.

3. Lower your chest toward the floor with your arms and elbows pointing away from your body. Push up, so that your arms are straight but your elbows aren't completely locked.

4. Squeeze your glutes and brace your abdominals throughout the pushup. Do not allow your lower back to sag or your hips to pike upward during the downward phase.

Modified Pushup

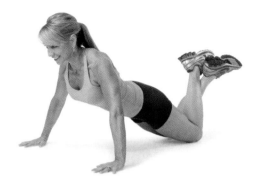

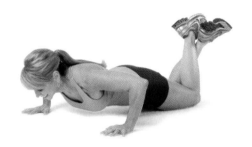

1. Get on your hands and knees, with your hands slightly wider than shoulder-width apart and in line with your chest. Cross your feet at the ankles, creating a straight line from the top of your head to your knees.

2. Keep your body as straight as possible, with your eyes focused straight down and your neck in a neutral position.

3. Lower your chest toward the floor with your arms and elbows pointing away from your body.

4. Push up, so that your arms are straight but your elbows aren't completely locked.

5. Squeeze your glutes and brace your abdominals throughout the pushup. Do not allow your lower back to sag or your hips to pike upward during the downward phase.

Pushup Incline

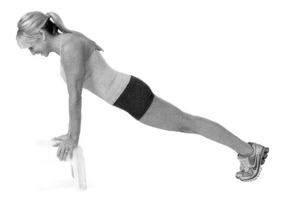

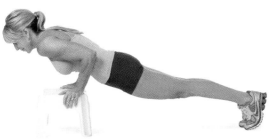

1. Get on your knees next to a step or stair. Place your hands shoulder-width apart on the step or stair. Get up on your toes.

2. Keep your body as straight as possible, with your eyes focused straight down and your neck in a neutral position.

3. Lower your chest toward the step or stair. Keep your arms close to your sides and your elbows pointing straight back.

4. Squeeze your glutes and brace your abdominals throughout the pushup. Do not allow your lower back to sag or your hips to pike upward during the downward phase.

Pushup Decline

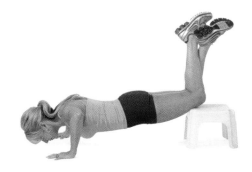

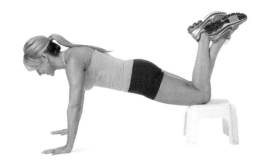

1. Put your knees on a step or stair, crossing your feet at the ankles.

2. Assume the pushup position, placing your hands shoulder-width apart on the floor in front of you.

3. Slowly lower your chest toward the floor. Keep your arms close to your sides.

4. Push up, so that your arms are straight but not locked.

Stacked-Toe Pushup

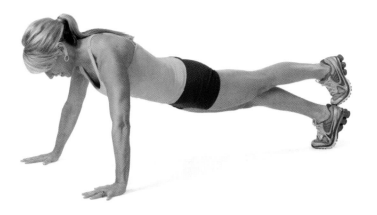

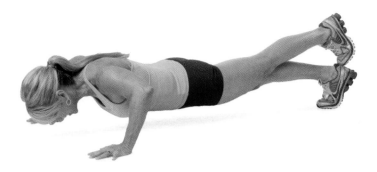

1. Start with your hands slightly wider than shoulder-width apart and in line with your chest.

2. Straighten your legs and place the toes of one foot on the heel of the foot on the floor. Keep your legs straight.

3. Lower your chest toward the floor with your arms and elbows pointing away from your body.

4. Push up, so that your arms are straight but your elbows aren't completely locked.

5. Squeeze your glutes and brace your abdominals throughout the pushup. Do not allow your lower back to sag or your hips to pike upward during the downward phase.

6. Change foot position and repeat the series.

Pushup Alternating Leg Lift

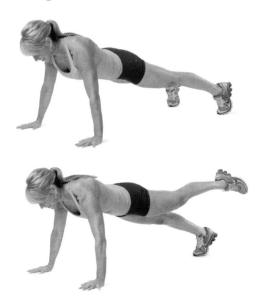

1. Lie face down on your mat with your hands slightly wider than shoulder-width apart and under your chest. Keep your fingers straight and your legs straight and slightly apart with your toes supporting your feet. Your weight should be on your hands and toes.

2. Keep your body as straight as possible, with your eyes focused straight down and your neck in a neutral position.

3. Extend your left hip to lift your left leg off the floor, keeping your knee straight.

4. Lower your chest toward the floor with your arms and elbows pointing away from your body.

5. As you push up, lower the extended leg to the floor while you simultaneously lift the opposite leg.

6. Squeeze your glutes and brace your abdominals throughout the pushup. Do not allow your lower back to sag or your hips to pike upward during the downward phase.

7. Repeat, alternating legs.

Spider Pushup

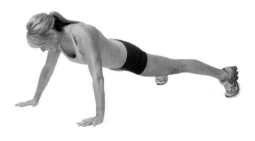

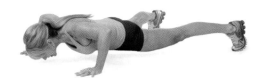

1. Start with your hands slightly wider than a regular pushup. Get up on your toes and place your feet as wide as it feels comfortable.

2. Keep your body as straight as possible, with your eyes focused straight down and your neck in a neutral position.

3. Lower your chest toward the floor with your arms and elbows pointing away from your body.

4. Push up so your arms are straight but your elbows aren't completely locked.

5. Squeeze your glutes and brace your abdominals throughout the pushup. Do not allow your lower back to sag or your hips to pike upward during the downward phase.

Elbow Plank to Pike

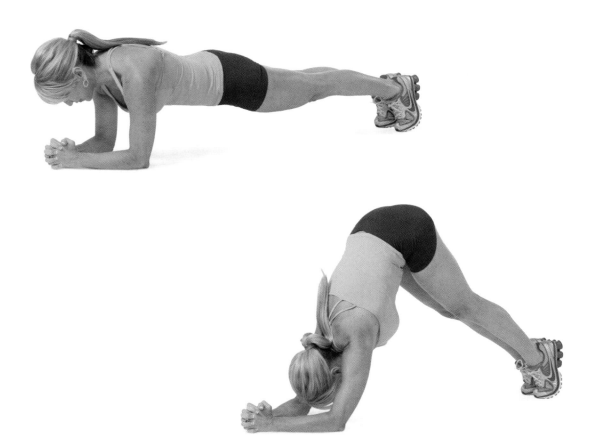

1. Place your feet shoulder-width apart and get on your toes. Rest your forearms on the floor and clasp your hands, creating a triangle.

2. Keep your body as straight as possible, with your eyes focused straight down and your neck in a neutral position when in the plank position.

3. Pike your hips toward the ceiling, keeping your head in alignment with your torso. Your feet will slide forward as you pike.

4. Lower and return to the starting position. Do not allow your lower back to sag during the downward phase.

Pushup to Side Plank

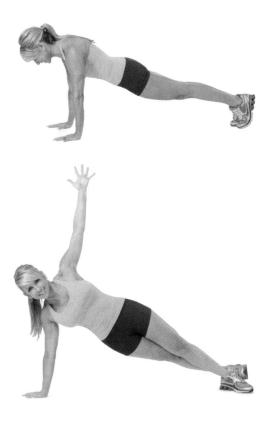

1. Start with your hands slightly wider than shoulder-width apart. Get up on your toes.

2. Keep your body as straight as possible, with your eyes focused straight down and your neck in a neutral position.

3. Lower your chest toward the floor with your arms and elbows pointing away from your body.

4. As you come up, shift your weight to the left side of your body and arm and rotate your body to the side as you bring your right arm up toward the ceiling into a side plank.

5. Lower your arm and body to the floor for another pushup and plank to the other side.

Pushup Knee Tuck

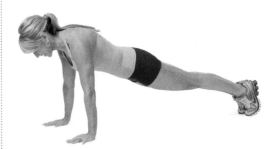

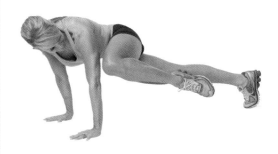

1. Start with your hands slightly wider than shoulder-width apart. Get up on your toes.

2. Keep your body as straight as possible, with your eyes focused straight down and your neck in a neutral position.

3. Lower your chest toward the floor as you simultaneously bend one knee toward the shoulder (same side).

4. Keep your hips parallel to the floor throughout the exercise. Avoid letting your hips or back pike upward or sag to the floor.

5. As you push up, straighten your bent knee and lower your leg to the floor.

6. Repeat, alternating knees.

Single Leg Pushup

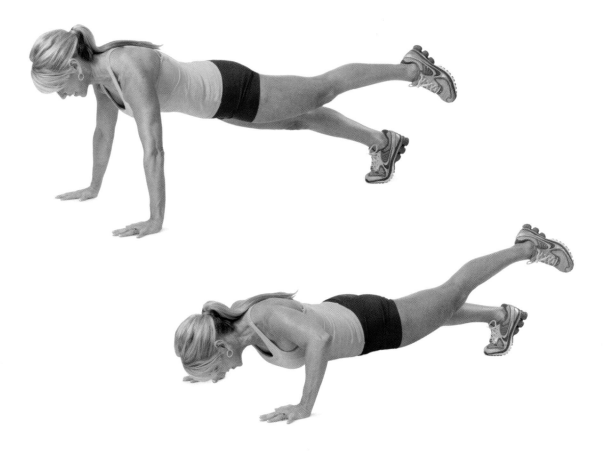

1. Start with your hands slightly wider than shoulder-width apart. Get up on your toes.

2. Keep your body as straight as possible, with your eyes focused straight down and your neck in a neutral position.

3. Extend your left hip to lift your left leg off the floor, keeping the knee straight.

4. Keep your leg elevated as you lift and lower your chest toward the floor, creating a straight line from the top of your head to your toe.

5. Squeeze your glutes and brace your abdominals throughout the pushup. Do not allow your lower back to sag or your hips to pike upward during the downward phase.

GET SERIOUS WITH THE PUSHUPS The moment you finish each exercise, drop and do your pushups! Do what you can, knowing that as you work your way through the circuit, each set of pushups will get tougher. That's the point, remember? We change your body by giving it a reason to change. When your arms are so tired you can barely finish the set of pushups, that's when you know you're doing it right!

I'm not gonna lie . . . pushups are not easy when you first start, but nothing is when you are learning. They'll get easier as you get stronger—and you *will* get stronger! You'll soon have so much pride in your pushup abilities, you'll want to perform 'em at cocktail parties!

Let's Go! The 5-Minute Warmup

You'll begin each circuit with the warmup below. You'll do it without weights—which will provide a rehearsal effect for your muscles for the exercises you're about to perform—but have a set of dumbbells nearby. You'll need them for the first exercise of your circuit.

To properly warm up, we need to pump blood through your large muscle groups and raise your core temperature. Nothing does that more effectively than the good old-fashioned squat. My goal is to help you do the squats with exceptional form so that your knees get stronger and your legs get leaner! Remember, focus on form, and slow is the way to go! Here are a few tips to keep in mind.

- Begin with feet shoulder-width apart.
- Transfer weight from the balls of your feet to your heels.
- Begin as if you are about to sit, pushing your hips back, bending your knees.
- Work to keep your shoulders back and chest up, but don't expect to be able to keep your back at a 90-degree angle.
- It's okay if your knees slide forward slightly, but work to keep them over your ankles.
- Slide both arms out in front of you, arms straight, at chest height to counterbalance your hips.
- If you feel you are about to tip over backward, you're probably doing this right.

Spinal Flex

8 REPS

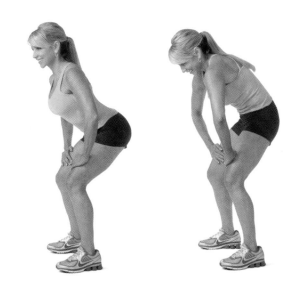

Squat

8 REPS

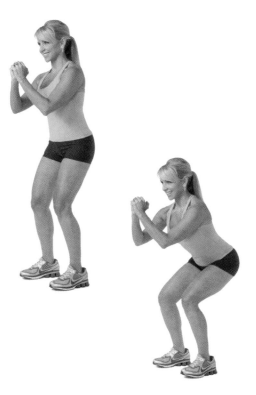

1. Begin with several shallow squats, as described above.

2. With each rep, increase the range of motion and squat deeper.

Body Weight Squat
Knee Lift, Alternating

8 REPS

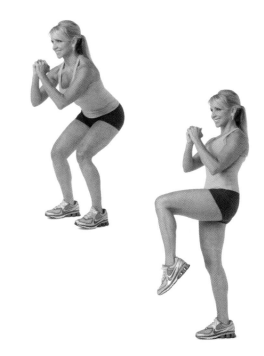

1. Squat to your lowest range—your arms in front at chest height.

2. As you begin to stand, draw one knee up toward your belly button as you pull your arm back.

3. Repeat, alternating knees.

Body Weight
Sumo Squat

8 REPS

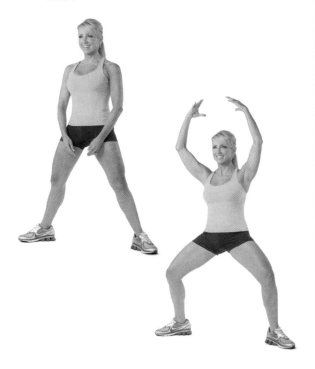

1. Position your feet wider than your shoulders.

2. Turn your toes out.

3. Lower your hips, bending your knees, maintaining an upright posture.

4. Imagine you are sliding your back down a wall.

5. As you rise up, perform a bicep curl (no weight, of course).

6. Tighten and engage the biceps as you flex upward.

7. Press your thighs forward, engaging the inner thighs and glutes as you lift.

8. Keep the knees soft.

Leg Lunge/Arm
Triceps Extensions

4 REPS

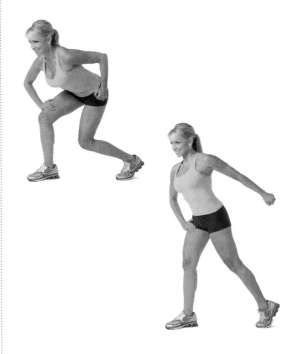

1. Transfer your weight to the heel of your forward leg.

2. Bend the left elbow, drawing it back past your ribs, and flexing to 90 degrees.

3. Lower your body as you flex your knee, maintaining weight on the forward leg, elbow above your back, fist at your rib cage.

4. As you begin to rise up, fully extend the elbow, flexing the back of your arm (triceps).

5. To keep your weight over the forward heel, your chest may lower slightly toward the thigh (no problem!).

6. Repeat on the other side.

Leg Lunge/Arm Triceps Extension/ Shoulder Circumduction

4 REPS

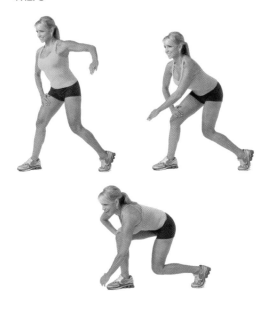

1. Transfer your weight to the heel of your forward leg.

2. Bend the left elbow, drawing it back past your ribs, and flexing to 90 degrees.

3. Lower your body as you flex your knee, maintaining weight on the forward leg, elbow above your back, fist at your rib cage.

4. As you begin to rise up, fully extend the elbow, flexing the back of your arm/triceps (repeat 4 times).

5. Continue lunging, slowly circling the shoulder with your arm fully extended (repeat 4 times).

6. To keep your weight over the forward heel, your ribs may lower slightly toward the thigh; keep your shoulders back.

7. Repeat on the other side.

Alternating Side Lunge— Shoulder Drops

4 REPS PER SIDE

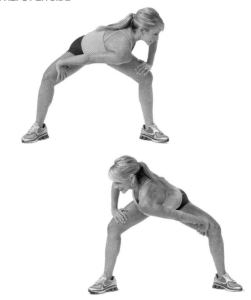

1. Face center with your feet slightly wider than a shoulder-width apart.

2. Bend the knees, placing your hands on your thighs.

3. As you lunge to the right, press the left shoulder toward the midline of your body. As you lunge to the left, press the right shoulder toward your midline.

4. Alternate lunging side to side.

Now that you've warmed up your muscles, you're ready to hit the circuit. If it takes you a little longer to warm up or you have soreness in one particular area, go ahead and spend a few more minutes warming up and doing gentle rhythmic stretching. The warmer your muscles, the better they'll perform!

Circuit 1

I use 15-pound dumbbells for most of these exercises, but match the weights you choose to your level of fitness. Momentary muscle-fatigue-induced failure should occur between the 10th and 12th rep. If you feel as though you could do a few more reps after 12, consider using a heavier weight for your next workout.

5-Minute Warmup (pages 225–228)

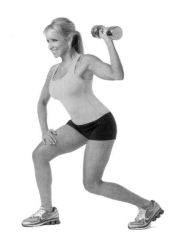

Lunge and Press

1. Stand with your feet shoulder-width or farther apart, hold a weight at shoulder height.

2. Take a very long step forward, landing with your weight on the heel of your forward foot.

3. Lower your body down until the front knee reaches nearly 90 degrees (modify as needed).

4. While in the lowest part of your lunge, press the weight overhead slowly (counting to 4).

5. While still in your low lunge, slowly lower the weight to shoulder height (counting to 4).

6. Next, by pushing off with the forward heel, step back to your starting position.

7. Repeat, alternating lunges for a total of 6 lunges and 12 overhead presses.

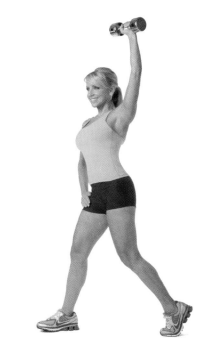

Pick Any Pushup
(pages 216–224)
1 SET (UP TO 12 REPS)

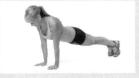
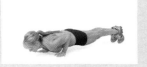

Alternating Bowler's Lunge/ Bicep Curl

1. Stand with your feet shoulder-width apart, one dumbbell in one hand.

2. Keep your elbows at your side, weights in the upward starting position of your bicep curl.

3. Transfer your weight to the left foot, then cross the right leg behind the left (as a bowler would when releasing the ball).

4. The majority of your weight should be on the forward leg.

5. Bend your forward knee and lower down, as if to lunge.

6. As you lower, press your left hip toward the left side of the room (tighten and engage the left glute).

7. While in your low lunge, engage the abs, and slowly lower the arm holding the dumbbell to full extension, then lift your arm to its starting position.

8. Now slowing return to a standing position.

9. Repeat, 6 lunge/bicep curls with one arm, then switch and repeat with the other arm.

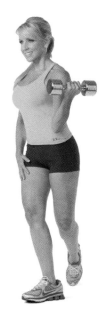

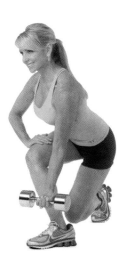

Pick Any Pushup
(pages 216–224)
1 SET (UP TO 12 REPS)

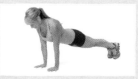

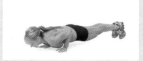

Inner Thigh Squat/
Overhead Press

1. Position your feet a little wider than shoulder-width apart, one dumbbell in each hand.

2. Turn your toes out.

3. Lower your hips, bending your knees and maintaining an upright posture.

4. Imagine you are sliding your back down a wall.

5. As you rise up, bend the elbow to perform a non-weighted bicep curl.

6. Tighten and engage the biceps as you flex upward.

7. Press your thighs forward, engaging the inner thighs and glutes as you lift.

8. Keep the knees soft.

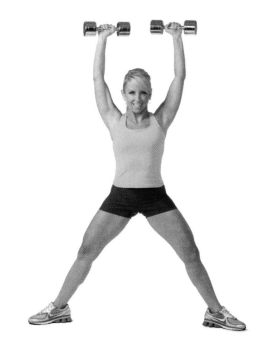

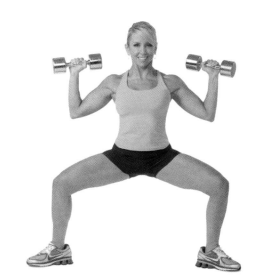

Pick Any Pushup
(pages 216–224)
1 SET (UP TO 12 REPS)

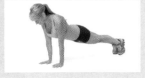

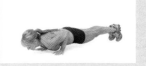

Squat/Hammer

1. Begin with your feet shoulder-width apart, weights by your side.

2. Transfer your weight from the balls of your feet to your heels, then squat slowly.

3. As you sit back into the squat, allow your weights to counterbalance your hips' pushing backward.

4. Slowly stand up and repeat.

5. Now standing, slowly lower the weights back to near full extension in front of your thighs.

6. Keep the biceps contracted and flexed throughout the exercise.

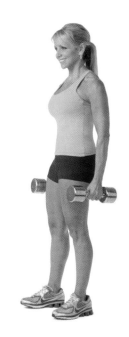

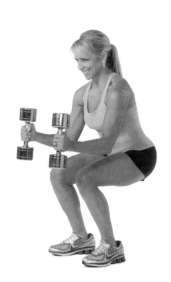

Pick Any Pushup
(pages 216–224)
1 SET (UP TO 12 REPS)

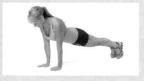

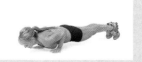

Bowler's Lunge/ Single-Arm Shoulder Press

1. Stand with your feet shoulder-width apart, one dumbbell in each hand.

2. Begin with the weights in an upward position, palms toward your face at about chin height.

3. Transfer your weight to the left foot, then cross the right leg behind the left (as a bowler would when releasing the ball).

4. The majority of your weight should be on the forward leg.

5. Bend your forward knee and lower down, as if to lunge.

6. As you lower, press your left hip toward the left side of the room (tighten and engage the left glute).

7. Slowly stand up, engaging the abs, and press the weight in your left hand overhead as you rotate the palm forward.

8. Lower the weight to start position and switch legs.

9. Repeat, alternating lunges for a total of 6 lunges and 12 overhead presses.

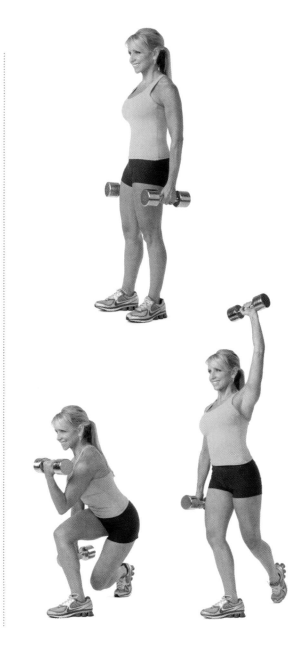

Pick Any Pushup
(pages 216–224)
1 SET (UP TO 12 REPS)

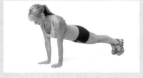 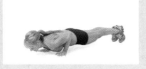

Reverse Lunge/
Bicep Curl

1. Stand with your feet shoulder-width or farther apart, pressing elbows into your waistline, weights up, biceps flexed.

2. Take a very long step back, keep your weight on the heel of your forward foot.

3. Lower your body down until the front knee reaches nearly 90 degrees (modify as needed).

4. While in the lowest part of your lunge, slowly lower the bicep curl (counting to 4).

5. While still in your low lunge, slowly flex and curl the weight back to the starting position (counting to 4).

6. Next, by pushing off with the forward heel, step back to your starting position.

7. To really get the most out of this exercise, stop the bicep curl about 4 inches from your shoulder.

8. Repeat, alternating lunges for a total of 6 lunges and 12 bicep curls.

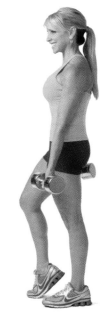

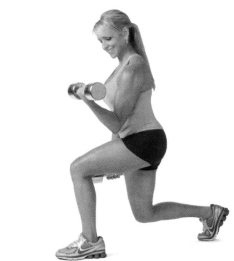

Pick Any Pushup
(pages 216–224)
1 SET (UP TO 12 REPS)

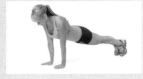
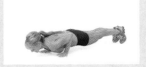

Circuit 2

I use 12-pound dumbbells for most of these exercises, but match the weights you choose to your level of fitness. Momentary muscle-fatigue-induced failure should occur between the 10th and 12th rep. If you feel as though you could do a few more reps after 12, consider using a heavier weight for your next workout.

5-Minute Warmup (pages 225–228)

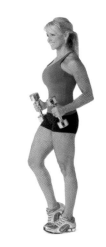

Lunge and Double Triceps Kick-Back

1. Stand with your feet shoulder-width or farther apart, holding weights at the front of your shoulder.

2. Take a very long step forward, landing with your weight on the heel of your forward foot.

3. Lower your body down until the front knee reaches nearly 90 degrees (modify as needed).

4. While in the lowest part of your lunge, hinge forward, drawing your elbow up toward the ceiling.

5. While in your lunge and hinged forward, extend the elbow (counting to 4).

6. While still in your low lunge, slowly lower the weight, your elbow joint at 90 degrees (counting to 4).

7. Next, by pushing off with the forward heel, step back to your starting position.

8. Repeat, alternating lunges for a total of 6 lunges and 12 triceps kick-backs.

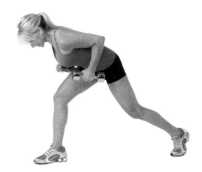

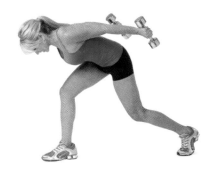

Pick Any Pushup
(pages 216–224)
1 SET (UP TO 12 REPS)

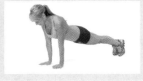
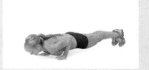

Alternating Bowler's Lunge—Medial Deltoid Raise

1. Stand with your feet shoulder-width apart, one dumbbell in each hand, arms resting at your sides, elbow slightly bent.

2. Transfer your weight to the left foot, then cross the right leg behind the left (as a bowler would when releasing the ball).

3. The majority of your weight should be on the front leg.

4. Bend your forward knee and lower down, as if to lunge (now nearly balancing on your front leg).

5. As you lower, press your left hip toward the left side of the room (tighten and engage the left glute).

6. While in your low lunge, engage the abs and slowly raise your arm to shoulder height, weights and elbows parallel to the floor.

7. While still in your lowest position, slowly lower the weights back to your side.

8. As you lift up, cross the opposite leg behind, as this exercise alternates legs.

9. Avoid shrugging your shoulders, swinging the weights, or leading with the weights.

10. Your knuckles, weights, and elbow should all line up parallel to the floor at the top of your rep.

11. Repeat, alternating lunges for a total of 6 lunges and 12 medial deltoid raises.

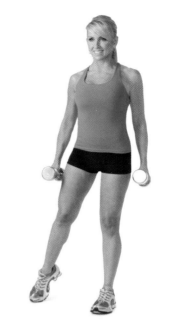

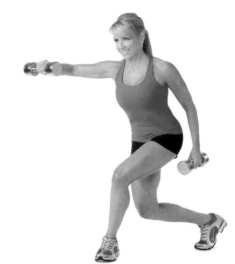

Pick Any Pushup
(pages 216–224)
1 SET (UP TO 12 REPS)

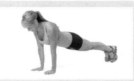
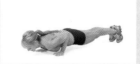

Squat with Overhead Triceps Extension

I use 10-pound dumbbells for this exercise.

1. Begin with your feet shoulder-width apart, with a weight cupped with both hands.

2. The weight should be held in front of you at chin height, with your elbows bent to 90 degrees if possible.

3. Transfer your weight from the balls of your feet to your heels, then squat slowly.

4. As you sit back into the squat, allow your weight to counterbalance your hips' pushing backward.

5. Slowly stand as you simultaneously push the weight overhead, then with your elbows tight to your head, flex or bend your elbows, lowering your weight behind your head to the back of your neck.

6. Now standing, slowly lift the weight back up, then lower to the flexed elbow position at chin height.

7. Repeat 12 times.

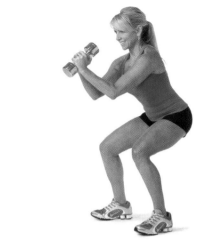

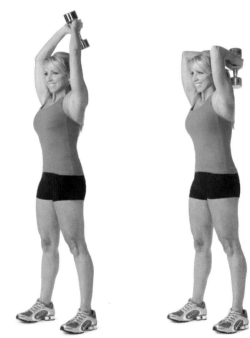

Pick Any Pushup
(pages 216–224)
1 SET (UP TO 12 REPS)

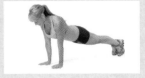
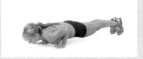

Inner Thigh Squat—Medial Deltoid Raise

1. Position your feet wider than shoulder-width apart (the wider stance is better for your knees), one dumbbell in each hand, arms resting at your sides, elbows slightly bent.

2. Turn your toes out.

3. Lower your hips, bending your knees and maintaining an upright posture.

4. Imagine you are sliding your back down a wall.

5. While in your low squat position, engage the abs and slowly raise your arms to shoulder height, weights and elbows parallel to the floor.

6. While still in your lowest position, push the thighs forward to engage the inner thighs, then lower the weights back to your side but avoid resting them on your thighs.

7. Avoid shrugging your shoulders.

8. Your knuckles, weights, and elbows should all line up parallel to the floor at the top of your rep.

9. Think of pushing your inner thighs toward the front of the room isometrically as you lift up.

10. Repeat 12 times.

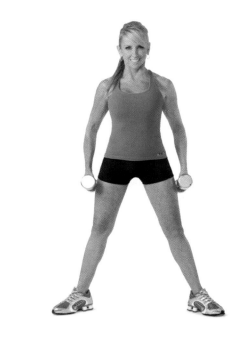

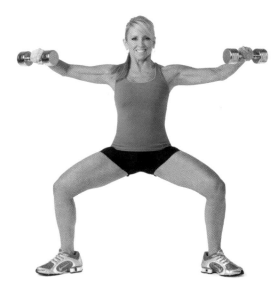

Pick Any Pushup
(pages 216–224)
1 SET (UP TO 12 REPS)

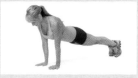 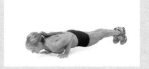

Reverse Runner's Lunge—Medial Deltoid Raise

1. Stand with your feet shoulder-width or farther apart, weights resting at your sides.

2. Take a very long step back, keeping your weight on the heel of your forward foot and dropping into a runner's lunge.

3. This exercise can be modified by simply keeping your lunge shallow (don't go so deep!).

4. Lower your body down until the front knee reaches 90 degrees or more (modify as needed).

5. While in the lowest part of your lunge, slowly raise your arm upward to shoulder height (counting to 4).

6. While still in your low lunge, slowly lower the weights to your sides, keeping the neck relaxed (counting to 4).

7. Next, by pushing off with the forward heel, step back to your starting position, then switch legs.

8. To really get the most out of this exercise, your palms should face downward and your elbows should be slightly bent.

9. Repeat, alternating lunges for a total of 6 lunges and 12 lateral raises.

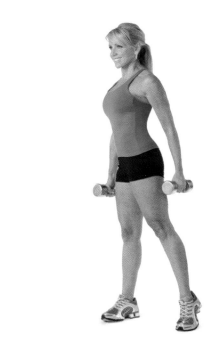

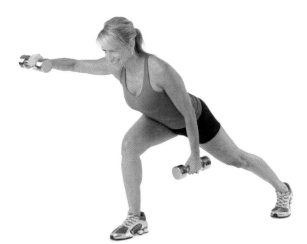

Pick Any Pushup
(pages 216–224)
1 SET (UP TO 12 REPS)

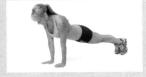

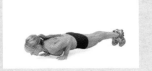

Plank Alternating Triceps Extension

1. Begin in a pushup position (also known as the plank); to modify, lower one knee.

2. Both weights can rest on the floor, just outside your hand position.

3. While in plank, grab one weight, flex the elbow to 90 degrees, and draw the elbow above your back.

4. With your elbow above the level of your back, fully extend, pressing your palm toward the sky.

5. While still in plank, flex or bend the arm and then lower the weight to the floor.

6. Repeat on the other side.

7. Continue alternating triceps extensions while holding this plank position.

8. Should your core or supporting arm tire, just lower one knee for a rep, then try to return to your toes as soon as you regain your strength.

9. Repeat, alternating triceps extensions for a total of 12.

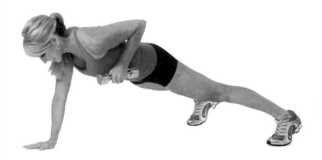

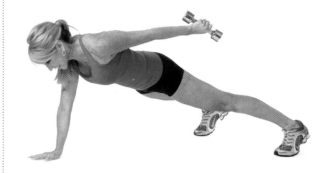

Pick Any Pushup
(pages 216–224)
1 SET (UP TO 12 REPS)

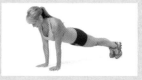
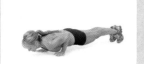

Circuit 3

I use 20-pound dumbbells for most of these exercises, except where indicated, but match the weights you choose to your level of fitness. Momentary muscle-fatigue-induced failure should occur between the 10th and 12th rep. If you feel as though you could do a few more reps after 12, consider using a heavier weight for your next workout.

5-Minute Warmup (pages 225–228)

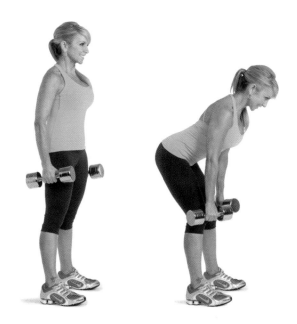

Straight Leg Deadlift/ Double Row

The effectiveness of this exercise depends upon maintaining a naturally arched or "flat back" spine. Avoid rounding your spine!

1. Stand with your feet shoulder-width apart (slightly wider than shoulder-width apart if your hamstrings are very tight).

2. Bend or hinge forward from the hip joint while maintaining a "soft" or slightly bent knee.

3. Keep your weights as close to your body as possible as you fold to nearly 90 degrees or parallel to the floor.

4. Once you feel the shoulder blades touch, continue pulling your elbows back until the weights are next to your rib cage.

5. Slowly extend the weights back down, as if sliding them down your thighs.

6. Continue to maintain a neutral spine as you return your torso to an upright position.

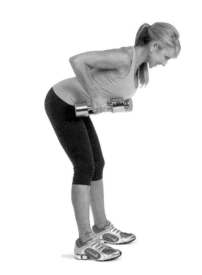

Pick Any Pushup
(pages 216–224)
1 SET (UP TO 12 REPS)

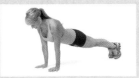
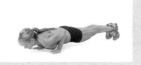

Single Leg Adduction/Bilateral Chest Fly

Working in opposition forces you to keep your abs engaged and work your core! To make this move more challenging, don't bring the arm or the leg all the way up. Instead, work in the bottom 50 percent of your range of motion.

1. Lie on your back, then press the weight above the midline of your body, keeping your elbow slightly bent.

2. Your opposite leg begins in an upward position at 90 degrees with the foot rotated out slightly.

3. As you lower the weight to the floor, maintain the same angle at your elbow (a slight bend) and lower your foot to just above the floor.

4. Slowly return to the upward position with both the foot and the single arm chest fly.

5. Complete 12 to 15 reps on one side, then switch.

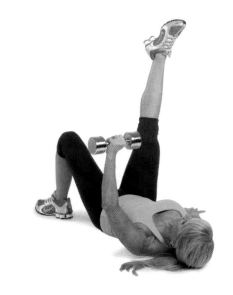

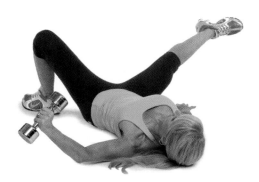

Pick Any Pushup
(pages 216–224)
1 SET (UP TO 12 REPS)

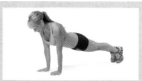
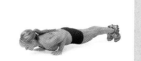

Lunge and Double Row

1. Stand with your feet shoulder-width apart, holding the weights at your hips.

2. Take a long step forward, landing with your weight on the heel of the forward foot.

3. Lower your body down until the front knee reaches nearly 90 degrees (modify as needed).

4. While in the lowest part of your lunge, hinge forward, then lower both weights to full extension toward the floor.

5. While still in your lunge and hinged forward, slowly draw the elbows back until the weights align with your rib cage (count to 4).

6. While still in your low lunge, slowly lower the weights (count to 4).

7. Step back to the starting position by pushing off with the forward heel.

8. Repeat, alternating lunges for a total of 6 lunges and 12 rows.

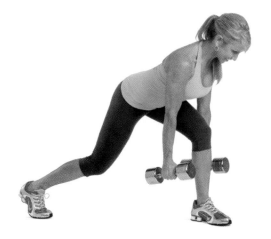

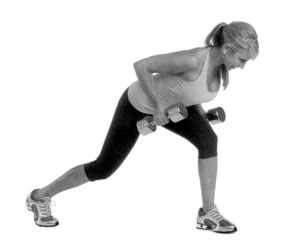

Pick This Pushup
INCLINE (PAGE 219)

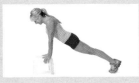
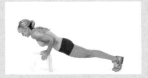

Alternating Bowler's Lunge/ Bent-Over Row

1. Stand with feet shoulder-width apart, a dumbbell in each hand and a slight bend in your elbows.

2. Transfer your weight to the left foot, then cross the right leg behind the left (as a bowler would when releasing the ball).

3. The majority of your weight should be on the heel of the forward leg.

4. Bend your forward knee and lower down, as if to lunge (now nearly balancing on your front leg).

5. As you lower, press your left hip toward the left side of the room (tighten and engage the left glute).

6. While in low lunge, engage the abs and slowly row both elbows back, keeping the elbows as close to your ribs as possible.

7. In this position, slowly lower the weights back to your side.

8. As you lift up, cross the opposite leg behind, as this exercise alternates legs.

9. Avoid shrugging your shoulders, swinging the weights, or leading with the weights.

10. Repeat, alternating lunges, for a total of 6 lunges and 12 rows.

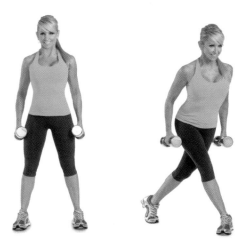
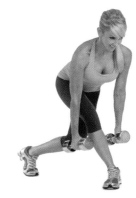
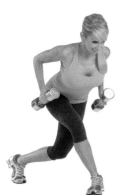

Pick This Pushup
DECLINE (PAGE 219)

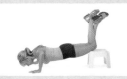
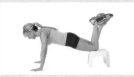

Chest Press/ Lower Abs

Warning: If you begin to feel your back arch up, you've gone too far! As you build strength, you'll be able to lower your legs even more.

1. Lie on your back, arms fully extended, one weight in each hand and pressed above you, near the midline of your body.

2. Cross your legs at the ankles and begin in an upward position at 90 degrees.

3. Begin by bending the elbows as you lower the weights.

4. As you lower the weight to the floor, take your feet to about 45 degrees.

5. Slowly return both the weights and your legs to the upward position.

6. To really target the lower abs, maintain a neutral spine and try to take your legs even lower.

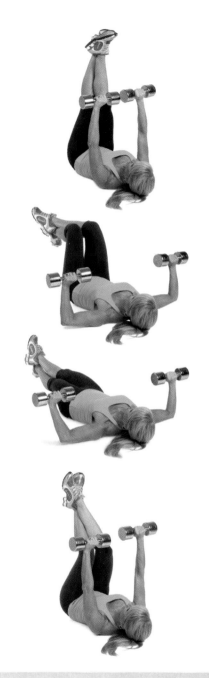

Pick This Pushup
PUSHUP TO SIDE PLANK (PAGE 223)

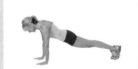 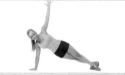

Low Lunge/Posterior Deltoid Row

6 TO 8 REPS PER LEG

1. Stand with your feet shoulder-width or farther apart, the weights resting at your side.

2. Take a very long step back, keeping your weight on the heel of your forward foot, and drop into a runner's lunge.

3. Lower your body down until the front knee reaches 90 degrees or more (modify as needed).

4. While in the lowest part of your lunge, draw the shoulders back with your knuckles facing the front of the room, elbows in the frontal plane, palms facing the back wall (not the floor).

5. While still in your low lunge, slowly lower the weights to your sides, keeping your neck relaxed.

6. Complete 6 reps per leg while staying in static lunge.

7. Pushing off with the forward heel, step back to the starting position to switch legs.

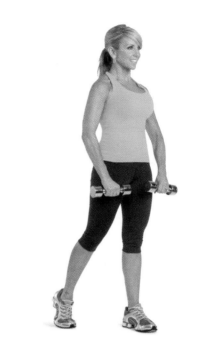

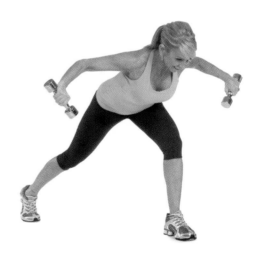

Stretch It Out

We are almost done! But before you hit the showers, take 5 more minutes that can make a world of difference in your progress.

Stretching improves muscle flexibility and joint mobility and decreases the likelihood of injury. By spending a few minutes stretching the muscles you've just worked, you will dramatically cut down on the soreness that is common 24 to 48 hours postworkout. Stretching while your muscles are warm also dramatically increases your overall flexibility and range of motion.

Think of your postworkout stretch as your exercise desert! Enjoy how good it feels to be done and to be taking a moment to release the lactic acid and tightness in your upper and lower body. Use this time to revel in your accomplishment and soothe tight muscles.

You can't make a mistake when it comes to stretching. Let the way you feel be your guide. Here are a few additional tips:

- Stretching immediately after your workout ensures that your muscles are warm and pliable.

- Concentrate on those muscles you used during your workout or circuit.

- Controlled stretching without bouncing is recommended for after your workout to prevent soreness.

- Hold each stretch for 15 to 60 seconds.

Remember, it takes only 5 minutes at the end of your workout to dramatically improve your recovery time and improve your results!

PART 3
THROW-AND-GO
RECIPES

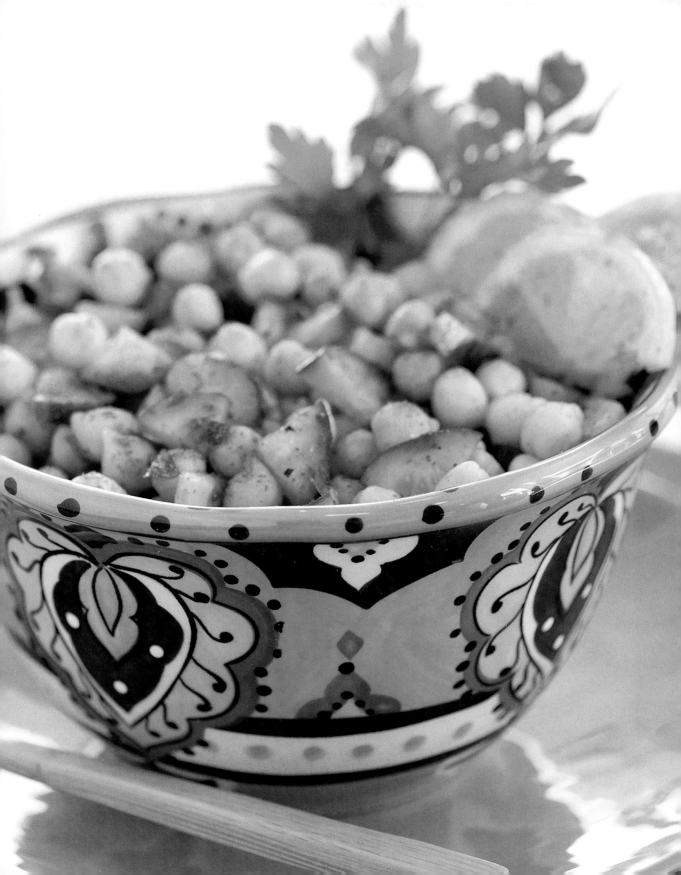

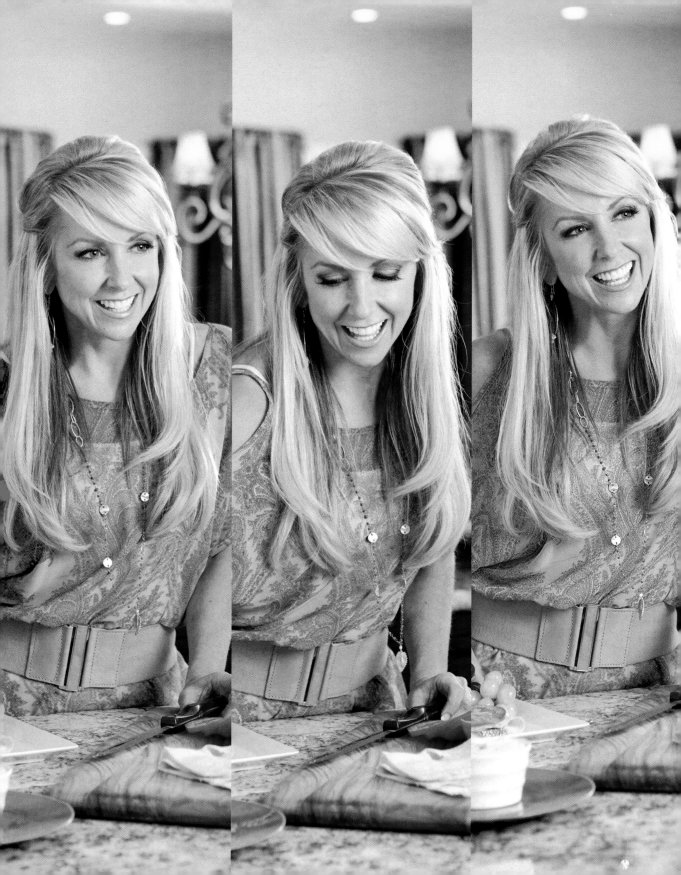

Throw-and-Go Is an Art Form!

It's one I've had to master out of necessity, resulting from life in the fast lane, a commitment to eating healthy, a love for food, and being challenged in the kitchen. Luckily, I married a guy who loves to cook. It's his hobby. He's really good at it, too! And certainly, if you own any of my exercise and weight-loss systems, you've probably tried many of his recipes. The truth is, the only time I get to eat those beautiful meals is when my personal chef (aka hubby) is available to cook for us. But nine times outta 10, he's flown out the door an hour before mealtime, as we run in opposite directions getting to meetings or appointments or transporting our kids to and from sporting events.

What I'm trying to say is, I'm not a nutritionist or a chef. If you're looking for amazing, mouthwatering fine cuisine with exotic ingredients, you can skip this chapter. You won't see any glossy pics of me grilling farm-fed salmon. Who in the heck has time to grow, harvest, cut, peel, clean and prepare an 18-ingredient healthy meal? Not me.

And I refuse to tell you what to eat and when to eat it. I don't care if you have egg white pancakes for dinner and chicken and brown rice for breakfast. Eat according to your cravings. If you're forcing yourself to eat something, you'll end up rebelling later, and that's not fair to your hips!

All that being said, these are my favorite Throw-and-Go Recipes. They're what I eat about 80 percent of the time, and I think you'll find that they mesh nicely with your on-the-move lifestyle.

I'm a small-meal kinda girl. I eat every 2½ or 3 hours. I love dessert, and I look forward most to breakfast and lunch-type entrees. That's reflected in my Throw-and-Go options!

Truth: I eat the same "concoctions" for five out of my six meals a day. Bret usually cooks the family something nice for dinner. If he's not around, I'll resort to whatever I'm craving from this selection. Some people like variety every day, at every meal. Not me. I eat the same menu every day for weeks and weeks and weeks until I never want to see it again.

I'll follow this pattern for months. Then often return to a Throw-and-Go option I grew tired of a year earlier. I've interviewed hundreds of forever-fit types and most say they do the same. Perhaps it's the predictability of your calorie consumption, or maybe it's the ease of preparation that comes when you have a Throw-and-Go memorized and no longer have to look at a recipe or weigh ingredients. I'm not sure why, but there's a real connection between this habit and the high number of forever-fit types I've met over the years. As I always say, to be a fit person, adopt the habits of healthy people. So go ahead, eat the same thing day after day until you never want to see it again. Then move on!

In general, my Throw-and-Go Recipes are from the first and second tier of the food ladder. I've given you loads of shortcuts. Sure, you could purchase all of these ingredients fresh and organic. Of course you could use your oven instead of the microwave. Duh. The point of these delicious options is that they are *speedy*— from prep to plate in 5 minutes or less!

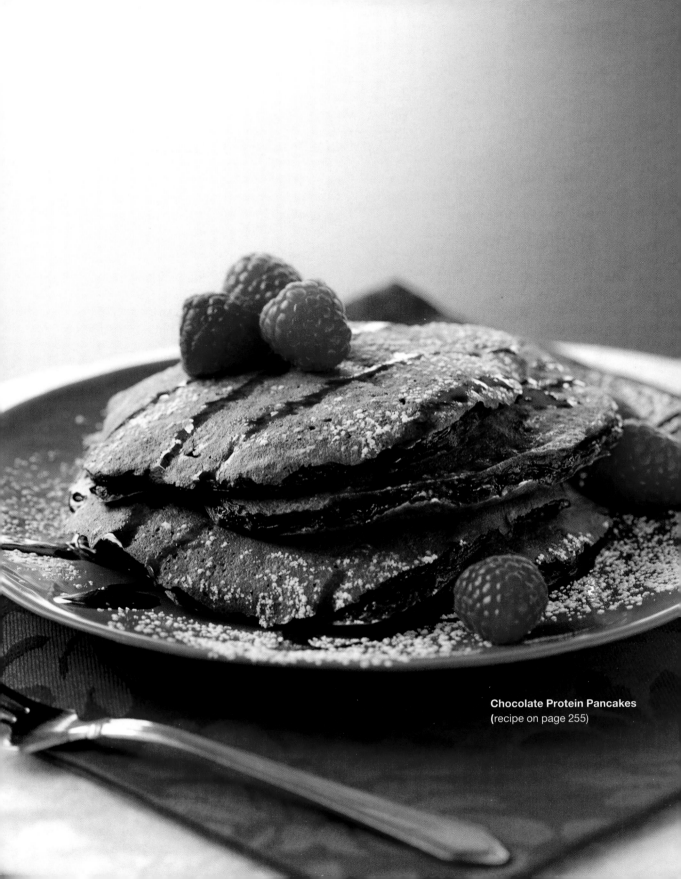

Chocolate Protein Pancakes
(recipe on page 255)

THE RECIPES

The Brands I Use and Love

First things first: Not every brand is available in every market. In fact, some of the items I've listed below I learned of not via a trip to the market but through a tight-knit group of supportive friends on Facebook! Social media is a great place to learn about new products and brands that haven't made their way to the big retailers' shelves but that calorie-conscious folks love to share among themselves.

Several of these brands I order from in bulk from the manufacturers' Web sites. They are staples! And now, like a secret handshake, I share them with you!

Peanut Butter

PB2 Powdered Peanut Butter. Powdered peanuts with a touch of salt, and that's it! You mix it with a little water to form a peanut butter paste (which does not taste much like the real deal, if you ask me). However, for recipes, desserts and protein shakes . . . two words: *I Die!!!* It's the bomb! Totally passes muster with most food police. You'll have to order this little number

(and the Chocolate PB2, below) directly from the manufacturer (www.bellplantation.com).

Chocolate PB2 Powdered Peanut Butter. It's the same as above, but with cocoa-bean powder. Peanut butter and chocolate—how could you not fall in love? Get to know me!

Better'n Peanut Butter. Much lower in fat and calories than traditional PB, but some all-natural added ingredients make the consistency a bit sticky (IMHO). I like it. My sister loves it. Is it the perfect food? No. But it's far better than loading up on all the fat from regular peanut butters. This one is available at most major grocery chains.

Naturally More. I love the taste and texture the flaxseeds add to this peanut butter. The best part is they've taken peanut butter and made it more than just a fatty spread with a little bit of protein. This recipe is enhanced with good stuff like omega-3 fatty acids, 25 percent more protein than most peanut butters, 50 percent more fiber, and far less fat! You can find it at most retailers and online at www.naturallymore.com.

Breads/Carbs

I gotta admit, even I—the everything in moderation girl—have been virtually scared straight of consuming carbs. Good carbs, bad carbs, complex and simple carbs: The bottom line is I like things that crunch, and there are days that I long for good old-fashioned bread.

Ezekiel 4:9 Organic Sprouted Bread. Delicious, but must be kept in the freezer.

110 calorie 100% whole wheat bagels. I call these skinny bagels. You can eat them toasted or not, but be prepared for an extracrunchy bagel if you do decide to toast them. Let's face it, they're not the thick, bready bagel you might be used to, but you need some options and this one is great!

Hummus

I dig hummus. Hummus alone is one thing, but on a sandwich or in a recipe it's about 10 thousand times better than fake mayo or even high-fat cheese. Buyer beware; not all hummus brands are created equal. I've done my research and I bring you the best!

Nasoya Super Hummus. This is the first and only hummus to deliver twice the protein and half the fat of the leading hummus brand. Look for it near tofu in the produce or dairy section of your food market.

Eggplant hummus. It's got half the fat and a surprisingly better taste, if you ask me!

Protein Shakes

Shakeology. There are bazillions of protein powders on the market. I never identified with any until this one came along. With only 140 calories per shake, and packed with the highest quality protein (18 grams per shake), this is my top pick because, truth be told, I'm not much of a veggie eater!

Shakeology is filled with the most extraordinary plants, fruits, nuts, and herbs—nature's secret weapons. Hundreds of doctors, scientists, and food experts have weighed in on these ingredients. Not cheap compared to the far less superior competitors, but very inexpensive when you factor in how much you would spend to pack the same nutrients into your daily diet. It tastes pretty good on its own, but to be honest, it's best doctored up with some the great recipes I've included here!

Tofu

Granted, some people are fully grossed out by tofu, my husband being one of them. When you prepare it correctly and use the right consistency, tofu is a fantabulous replacement for lean animal proteins. Tofu takes on the flavor of whatever its being prepared with. Maybe you just had a bad experience with the white tasteless curd-looking stuff. Put your big-girl panties on and try it again!

Trader Joe's High Protein Organic Tofu. I have no idea what Wonder Woman was eating to have that rockin' body, but I wouldn't be surprised if it was high-protein organic tofu. At 100 calories and 14 grams of protein, this concoction chameleon is dense with nutritional wonders and mega-low in carbs and fat.

Nasoya Organic Cubed Extra Firm Tofu. This brand is readily available and perfect for making vegetarian and vegan recipes. It's precut for convenience, so toss a healthy salad in no time! And check out our Healthy Tofu Pizza recipe on page 269.

Chocolate Protein Pancakes

Sometimes you want chocolate and bread. This is kinda the best of both worlds! I love to eat these pancakes warm with a few banana slices rolled in the center and little drizzle of honey. I love them cold, too, to dip into my favorite yogurt!

1 cup egg whites

1½ packets Quaker Oats Weight Control Maple & Brown Sugar Instant Oatmeal

1 teaspoon vanilla extract

1 teaspoon ground cinnamon

½ cup Chocolate Shakeology protein powder

Truvía sweetener, to taste (For this recipe, start with 3 small individual packets.)

Mix the eggs whites, oatmeal, vanilla, cinnamon, protein powder, and sweetener in a blender and process until completely blended.

Pour the batter in small medallions on a hot griddle or nonstick skillet. (They'll be a little thick, so use the back of a spoon to flatten them to about 4" in diameter.)

Flip once the edges start to bubble. Lightly brown on each side. Voilà! Chocolate pancakes.

MAKES 8

Per serving (1 pancake): 91 calories, 10 g protein, 12 g carbohydrates, 1 g total fat, 2 g dietary fiber, 105 mg sodium

Dairy-Free Orange 50/50

Technically speaking, this is a low-dairy recipe if you use a protein powder made from whey. Soy-based protein powders are harder to find, but they do exist! If you have only a slight sensitivity to dairy, I think you'll find this recipe works just fine, and if you close your eyes and think positive, it tastes a lot like a 50/50 bar with way more nutritional value.

1 scoop Greenberry Shakeology protein powder (or vanilla protein powder of your choice)

1 cup water

2 tablespoons fat-free, sugar-free cheesecake-flavored instant pudding mix

1 packet Crystal Light On the Go Sunrise Classic Orange drink mix, to taste

2 cups ice

Toss the protein powder, water, pudding mix, flavor packet, and ice into a blender. Blend away.

Pour into a glass and enjoy!

MAKES 1 SERVING

Per serving: 175 calories, 15 g protein, 25 g carbohydrates, 1 g total fat, 3 g dietary fiber, 414 mg sodium

Chocolate-Covered Strawberry Protein Shake

I love to start my day with a protein shake. This is so easy to make, it's ridiculous.

1 scoop chocolate protein powder

1 cup water

½ cup almond milk

½ cup frozen strawberries

Ice to taste

Toss the protein powder, water, milk, strawberries, and ice into your blender. Blend from medium speed to high. Pour into a glass and enjoy!

MAKES 1 SERVING

Per serving: 190 calories, 17 g protein, 26 g carbohydrates, 2 g total fat, 5 g dietary fiber, 86 mg sodium

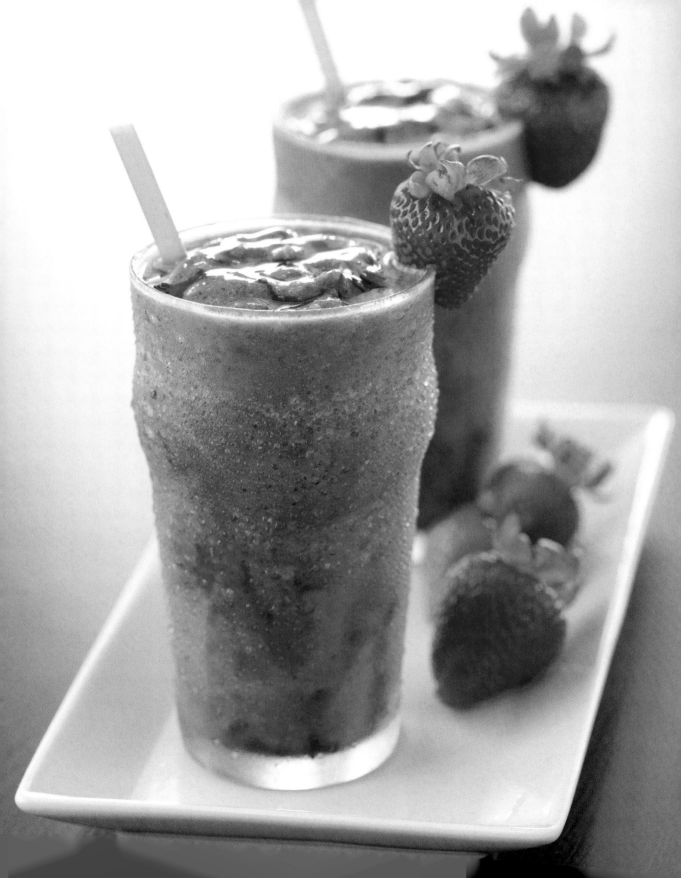

Protein-Packed Apple Surprise

This is a go-to breakfast for me! If the consistency of cottage cheese freaks you out, use fat-free Greek yogurt for even more protein. Don't do dairy? Make this with instant steel-cut oatmeal. Delish!

½ cup fat-free cottage cheese

Ground cinnamon, to taste

Truvía or Stevia sweetener, to taste

¼ cup walnuts

1 medium apple, diced

Throw the cottage cheese in a bowl. Add as much cinnamon and sweetener as you'd like. Mix.

Sprinkle in the walnuts and apple. Eat!

MAKES 1 SERVING

Per serving: 340 calories, 17 g protein, 40 g carbohydrates, 17 g total fat, 6 g dietary fiber, 432 mg sodium

Peanut Butter and Banana Wrap

I love this warm breakfast treat!

1 6-inch whole wheat low-carb tortilla

2 tablespoons PB2 powdered peanut butter mixed to taste, or organic peanut butter

½ banana, sliced

Microwave the tortilla for 10 seconds. Spread the peanut butter on the tortilla and add the bananas.

Roll and enjoy!

MAKES 1

Per serving: 148 calories (made with PB2) or 310 calories (made with full-calorie peanut butter), 13 g protein, 30 g carbohydrates, 18 g total fat, 11 g dietary fiber, 121 mg sodium

Spicy Egg White Scramble

A delicious alternative to a fat-packed omelet.

3 egg whites

1 slice turkey breast, chopped

¼ cup black beans, no salt added

2 tablespoons salsa

Heat a nonstick skillet coated with cooking spray over medium heat.

Add the egg whites and turkey breast. Cook for about 1 minute.

Add the black beans and salsa and heat until warm.

MAKES 1 SERVING

Per serving: 146 calories, 23 g protein, 12 g carbohydrates, 0.5 g total fat, 3 g dietary fiber, 308 mg sodium

High-Protein Breakfast Wrap

You can prepare this breakfast in minutes and it will keep you going for hours!

2 ounces cooked chicken, turkey, or tofu

3 egg whites

1 cup fresh spinach

1 slice reduced-fat cheese of your choice (Fat-free feta cheese is a great option.)

1 6-inch whole wheat tortilla

Heat a nonstick skillet coated with a cooking spray over medium heat.

Add the chicken, turkey, or tofu (your choice); egg whites; and spinach. Scramble together for about 5 minutes, until the eggs are thoroughly cooked.

Add the cheese and remove from the heat.

Pile the mixture into the tortilla, wrap it up, and love it!

MAKES 1

Per serving: Chicken Wrap: 305 calories, 39 g protein, 15 g carbohydrates, 9 g total fat, 9 g dietary fiber, 715 mg sodium; Turkey Wrap: 303 calories, 36 g protein, 30 g carbohydrates, 4 g total fat, 6 g dietary fiber, 988 mg sodium; Tofu Wrap: 325 calories, 32 g protein, 32 g carbohydrates, 8 g total fat, 7 g dietary fiber, 646 mg sodium

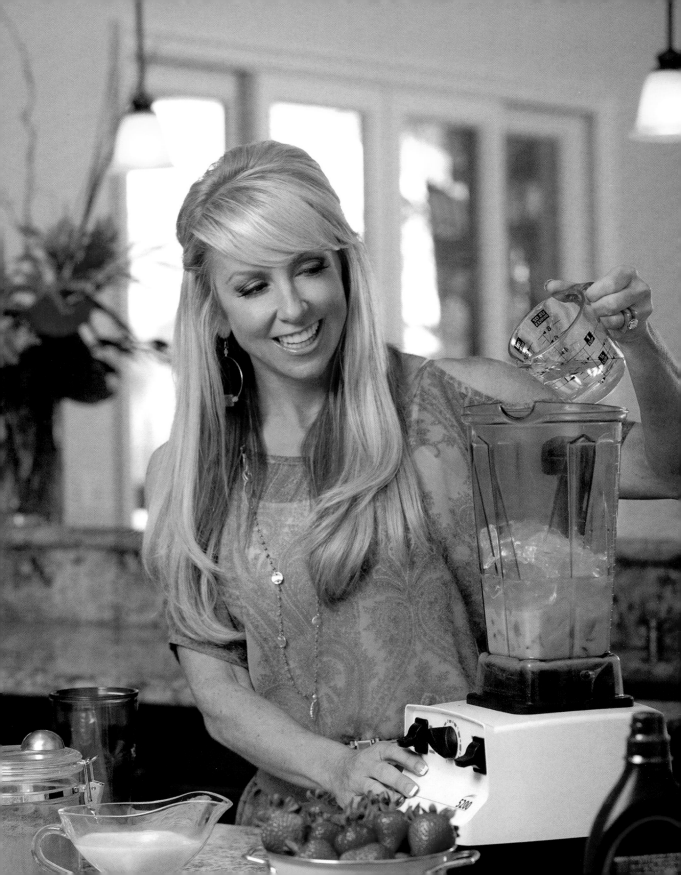

Minty Shamrock Protein Shake

If you're not using Greenberry Shakeology, you don't need to add the peanut butter. Greenberry is loaded with veggies and nutrient-dense ingredients. For some reason, the peanut butter completely "cuts" that "green" aftertaste. The PB is not needed if you will be making your shake with regular vanilla protein powder.

1 scoop Greenberry Shakeology protein powder (or a vanilla protein powder of your choice)

2 heaping tablespoons PB2 powdered peanut butter (or 1 teaspoon peanut butter)

2 tablespoons fat-free, sugar-free cheesecake-flavored instant pudding mix (This makes it creamy like ice cream.)

Couple of drops of mint extract (Play with the amount. Too much will clear your sinuses, and too little makes the shake blah.)

2 cups ice

Truvía or Stevia sweetener, to taste

Toss the protein powder, peanut butter, pudding mix, mint, ice, and sweetener into a blender. Blend from medium speed to high, adding water as needed until the shake has your preferred consistency.

Pour into a glass and enjoy!

MAKES 1 SERVING

Per serving: 210 calories, 20 g protein, 33 g carbohydrates, 2 g total fat, 5 g dietary fiber, 513 mg sodium

Egg White McLeanwich

This is wonderful on Ezekiel toast, too!

1 Thomas' Double Fiber Honey Wheat English Muffin

1 slice 97% lean honey ham

¼ cup egg whites

1 slice Kraft 2% American Cheese Single

Toast the English muffin.

In a skillet coated with cooking spray, warm the slice of ham over medium heat.

Remove and set aside the ham. Use the same small pan to cook the egg whites.

Place the ham and egg on the bottom half of the toasted muffin, then top with the cheese and the remaining muffin top. Off to work!

MAKES 1

Per serving: 182 calories, 17 g protein, 27 g carbohydrates, 1 g total fat, 5 g dietary fiber, 660 mg sodium

Super Hummus Deviled Eggs

Calories for 4 egg halves: 80 calories total. Crazy! They're so good! Go ahead and make 8 halves and count this as a meal! By the way, you'll go through egg whites like crazy—I probably eat 6 a day—so hard-cook a dozen eggs every Sunday night. Peel all of 'em when cool and place in a covered container in the fridge. Easy-peasy!

2 hard-cooked eggs (cooled)

2 tablespoons Nasoya Super Hummus

Peel the cooled eggs. Cut each egg in half and discard the yolk.

Replace the yolk with ½ tablespoon of hummus in each half.

MAKES 1 SERVING

Per serving: 84 calories, 11 g protein, 3 g carbohydrates, 3 g total fat, 1 dietary fiber, 231 mg sodium

Healthy Waldorf Salad

Triple this recipe to last you several meals. Chill and have it on hand for lunch or breakfast! Optional: Serve on romaine lettuce leaves.

- ¼ cup Fage Total 0% Plain Greek Yogurt (or your favorite fat-free Greek-style yogurt)
- ½ teaspoon orange juice or lemon juice
- 1 chicken breast
- ½ tart green apple, peeled, cored, and diced small
- 1 stalk celery, cut into small pieces (optional)
- ½ cup seedless grapes, halved
- ¼ cup dried cranberries or golden raisins
- 10 toasted raw almonds, slightly chopped

In a small bowl, whisk the yogurt and orange juice. Set aside.

In a skillet, bring 2 inches of water to a boil. Add the chicken, reduce the heat, and simmer for 8 to 10 minutes. *Do not let the chicken boil or it will get tough.*

Cool the chicken and cut into 1-inch chunks. Combine with the apple, celery (if using), grapes, dried cranberries or raisins, and almonds.

Give the yogurt mixture another stir; pour over the chicken and toss well to coat. Chill for at least 1 hour.

MAKES 2 SERVINGS

Per serving: 220 calories, 19 g protein, 26 g carbohydrates, 5 g total fat, 2 g dietary fiber, 94 mg sodium

Cucumber, Tomato and Basil Salad

This concoction is a staple for me!

- 1 medium cucumber
- 1 cup grape or cherry tomatoes
- 2 ounces low-fat part-skim mozzarella cheese, diced
- ¼ cup chopped fresh basil
- ½–1 teaspoon extra-light virgin olive oil
- Balsamic vinegar, to taste
- Ground black pepper to taste

Peel and chop the cucumber. Place in a bowl.

Add the tomatoes, cheese, and basil. Lightly drizzle with olive oil, vinegar, and pepper.

Toss and enjoy!

MAKES 1 SERVING

Per serving: 204 calories, 19 g protein, 17 g carbohydrates, 8 g total fat, 6 g dietary fiber, 408 mg sodium

Wilt-Free, Guilt-Free Salad with Feta, Raspberries, and Apples

My secret to using nuts in recipes: I buy the 100-calorie packs. When I want this salad, I take out a pack and pound those suckers into bite-size pieces right in the pack with whatever tool's handy. Who can ever find a mallet when she needs one? I've used a soup can to pound out my nuts!

1 Fuji apple

½ cup raspberries

½ cup blackberries

¼ cup crumbled reduced-fat feta cheese

3 cups any 3-lettuce prepackaged blend

1 cup fresh spinach

¼ cup crushed almonds

Dice up the apple. Don't worry about it being all cute.

Toss the apples, raspberries, blackberries, and feta into a small plastic sandwich bag. Throw your lettuce and spinach into a to-go container.

Wrap the nuts in a separate foil pouch to keep them crisp. (That's the secret to not having your salad get all wilted and keeping the crunch of your almonds.)

When you're ready to eat, sprinkle almonds on top. What about dressing? Between the cheese and the fruit, this salad is very moist and flavorful all by its lonesome. You can add some ground black pepper and/or low-fat dressing if you need to, but this salad is so flavorful without it, I think you can save yourself the unnecessary calories. Enjoy!

MAKES 1 SERVING

Per serving: 366 calories, 16 g protein, 48 g carbohydrates, 7 g total fat, 13 g dietary fiber, 517 mg sodium

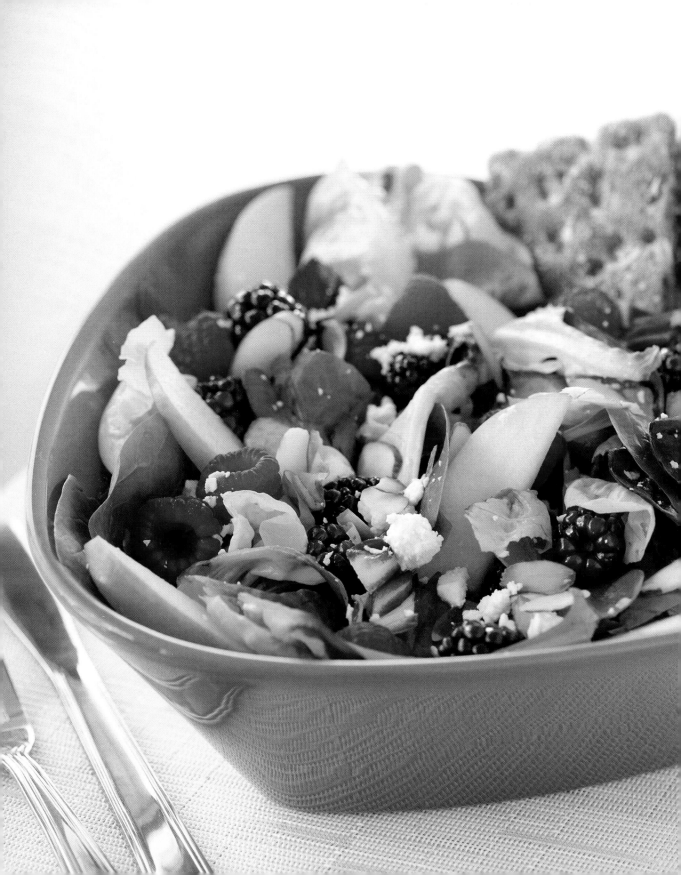

To-Die-For Hummus Quick Wrap

So simple, if you couldn't already tell from the ingredients.

1 6-inch low-carb tortilla (La Tortilla Factory is 50 calories, high fiber, high protein, low fat.)

2 tablespoons Nasoya Super Hummus

1 ounce fat-free feta cheese

1 ounce roasted red peppers (Feel free to used the canned variety.)

Toss your wrap or tortilla in the microwave, covered with a damp paper towel, for about 15 seconds, until it is warm and soft.

Plop the hummus on the wrap. Sprinkle on the feta and top with the roasted peppers. (My mouth is watering!)

Roll and go, baby, go!

MAKES 1

Per serving: 146 calories, 16 g protein, 16 g carbohydrates, 5 g total fat, 9 g dietary fiber, 717 mg sodium

Asian Tofu Brown Rice Bowl

If you have the time—and you probably will, because this whole concoction takes less than 2 minutes to make—chop up and add some carrots or throw in a few snow peas. Go for it!

½ cup Uncle Ben's Ready Rice Whole Grain Brown

1 teaspoon soy sauce

1 teaspoon sesame seeds

4 ounces Nasoya Organic Cubed Extra Firm Tofu

Nuke the pouch of rice in the microwave for 90 seconds. Measure out ½ cup. (Save the remaining ½ cup to use another day.)

In a small microwaveable bowl, mix the soy sauce, sesame seeds, and tofu. Microwave for about 45 seconds.

Pour over the brown rice.

MAKES 1 SERVING

Per serving: 269 calories, 18 g protein, 26 g carbohydrates, 11 g total fat, 3 g dietary fiber, 316 mg sodium

Chickpea Salad

If you want to get crazy, you can add a little bit of sliced avocados and some parsley to garnish. But it's *really* good just like this.

1 can (16 ounces) chickpeas, drained and rinsed

2 cloves garlic, pressed

½ cucumber, sliced or diced

1 tablespoon extra-virgin olive oil

Splash of lemon juice or white wine vinegar

Combine the chickpeas, garlic, cucumber, olive oil, and lemon juice or vinegar. Add salt and freshly ground black pepper to taste, mix well, and *mmm mmm!!*

MAKES 4 SERVINGS

Per serving: 97 calories, 3 g protein, 12 g carbohydrates, 4 g total fat, 3 g dietary fiber, 166 mg sodium

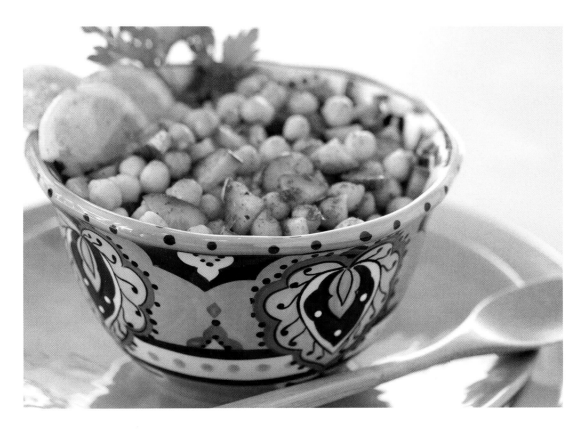

Bret's Turkey Chili

My hubby makes this special dish for me when it's cold outside. I mix the leftovers with egg whites for a morning scramble. This is the most popular recipe with all of my fans! People rave about it! It takes 5 minutes to make! (Don't believe me? Watch my video.)

- ½ medium onion, chopped
- 2 cloves garlic, chopped
- 1 pound lean ground turkey
- 1 package Lawry's Chili Seasoning
- 1 can (14.5 ounces) diced tomatoes
- 1 can (14.5 ounces) whole kernel corn
- 1 can (14.5 ounces) black beans
- 1 can (14.5 ounces) chili or pinto beans
- 1 tablespoon tomato paste

In a large saucepan coated with cooking spray, cook the onion and garlic until softened. Add the turkey and chili seasoning and cook until lightly browned.

Add the tomatoes, corn, beans, and tomato paste.

Cook on medium heat for 20 minutes, or add 1 cup water and simmer on low for hours for a really deliciously juicy chili!

MAKES 6 SERVINGS

Per serving (1 cup): 296 calories, 23 g protein, 37 g carbohydrates, 7 g total fat, 8 g dietary fiber, 1,097 mg sodium

5-Minute Creamy Fire-Roasted Chicken Salsa and Brown Rice

Get ready to look to the skies above and say, "Thank you, heaven, for the most delicious 5-minute meal I've ever had!"

- ½ cup Uncle Ben's Ready Rice Whole Grain Brown
- 2 tablespoons Fage Total 0% Plain Greek Yogurt (or your favorite fat-free Greek-style yogurt)
- ¼ cup fire-roasted salsa
- 4 ounces cooked skinless chicken breast, diced

Microwave a pouch of rice for 90 seconds; measure out ½ cup. (Save the remaining ½ cup to use another day.)

Place 1 tablespoon of the yogurt in a bowl. Add the rice and salsa and mix.

Meanwhile, toss the chicken into another bowl and warm in the microwave for about 40 seconds.

Throw the yogurt mix and chicken together and give it a good stir.

Want to make it creamier? Add that second tablespoon of yogurt. Need more fire? Add more salsa—it's basically a calorie freebie!

MAKES 1 SERVING

Per serving: 326 calories, 40 g protein, 24 g carbohydrates, 6 g total fat, 1 g dietary fiber, 457 mg sodium

Note: I often cook up 4 chicken breasts and multiply the recipe ingredients by 4. That is to say, 2 cups rice, ½ cup Greek yogurt, ½ cup salsa. That way, I make enough for 3 or 4 days all at once!

Healthy Tofu Pizza

Although this takes 50 minutes to bake, I still consider it a Throw-and-Go—so easy to just throw the ingredients on the whole wheat crust, and so worth the wait!

1 15-inch whole wheat pizza crust, unbaked

12½ ounces superfirm tofu

1 cup tomato sauce

¼ cup Parmesan cheese

2 scallions, sliced

1 cup sliced mushrooms

¾ cup diced green bell pepper

1½ cups mozzarella cheese, shredded

Preheat the oven to 350°F. Bake the pizza crust for 10 to 15 minutes.

In the meantime, crumble the tofu in a bowl. Mix in the tomato sauce and Parmesan.

When the crust is ready, evenly spread the tofu mixture on top. Sprinkle on the scallions, mushrooms, and pepper. Top with the mozzarella.

Bake for 10 to 15 minutes more until the crust is done and the cheese is melted.

MAKES 4–6 SERVINGS

Per serving: 300 calories, 20 g protein, 29 g carbohydrates, 13 g total fat, 6 g dietary fiber, 421 mg sodium

Low-Fat Veggie Mex Layered Dip with Cucumber "Chips"

This is 9-layer bean dip for fit people. Don't get all caught up in keeping the layers separate. Just throw all the ingredients into one bowl, then dip away! And trust me, you're gonna wanna double-dip those crunchy cuke slices. Since many of these ingredients come from a can, cover 'em in foil and experience this treat several times this week!

2 cucumbers

2 tablespoons fat-free refried beans

2 tablespoons fat-free chili

Salsa (as much as you want!)

2 tablespoons Fage Total 0% Plain Greek Yogurt (or fat-free sour cream, if you prefer)

¼ cup fat-free cheddar cheese

¼ cup diced tomatoes

¼ cup diced chile peppers

Black olives (optional)

Taco seasoning (optional)

Slice the cucumbers ¼ inch thick.

Place the beans, chili, salsa, yogurt, cheese, tomatoes, and peppers in a bowl. Stir. If you've got a few extra seconds, add a sprinkle of black olives and a dash of taco seasoning, if desired.

Chill for 2 hours if any ingredients were hot when you put them in. If not, go for it!

MAKES 1 SERVING

Per serving: 221 calories, 22 g protein, 34 g carbohydrates, 0.5 g total fat, 9 g dietary fiber, 848 mg sodium

Ezekiel Turkey, Hummus, Avocado Open-Face Sandwich

Ezekiel bread has no preservatives. That means if you don't eat the whole loaf within a few days of bringing it home, things start to grow. At my house, as soon as this bread comes home from the store, it goes straight into the freezer. I really eat Ezekiel only in toast form. I find it kinda dry otherwise, but it makes a supercrunchy, hearty, high-fiber toast. I learned about this bread from a bikini model in one of my classes!

1 slice Ezekiel bread, toasted

2 tablespoons Nasoya Super Hummus

2 slices lean turkey meat

1 slice tomato

¼ avocado, sliced or spread

Toast the bread. (Let it sit for a few minutes after toasting if you want it supercrunchy.)

Layer the bread first with hummus, then turkey. Add the tomato and top with the avocado. Get in my belly!

MAKES 1

Per serving: 252 calories, 21 g protein, 21 g carbohydrates, 9 g total fat, 7 g dietary fiber, 540 mg sodium

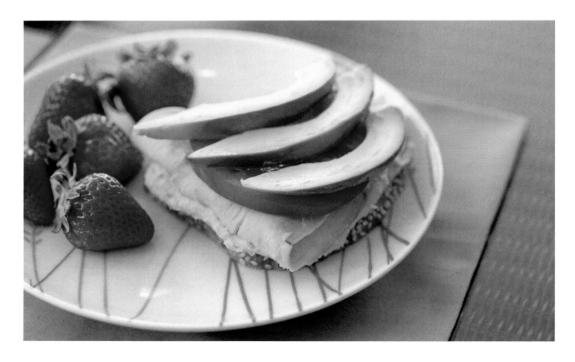

EZ Tomato-Basil Chicken

A go-to dinner made up of two ingredients. Can you say throw and go?!

½ of a 28-ounce can (about 1½ cups) crushed tomatoes with added basil

1 pound boneless, skinless chicken breast tenders

Preheat the oven to 350°F.

Pour half of the tomatoes (¼ of the can) into a medium baking pan. Lay the chicken in the pan. Pour the rest of the tomatoes (another ¼ of the can) evenly over the chicken.

Bake for about 30 minutes, until the chicken is cooked through.

Allow the chicken to cool and the sauce to thicken slightly before serving. Ta-da!

MAKES 4 SERVINGS

Per serving: 140 calories, 27 g protein, 7 g carbohydrates, 0.5 g total fat, 1 g dietary fiber, 340 mg sodium

Seared Tofu and Cucumbers

Tofu is an awesome source of protein. This works great if you marinate it a few hours ahead of making it.

7 ounces firm tofu

Thai peanut sauce (homemade or store bought)

Fresh spinach

½ medium cucumber, sliced

Chop the tofu into small cubes. Wrap in two paper towels and place something heavy on top for 10 to 15 minutes, until most of the water is drained from the tofu.

Place the tofu in a bowl and pour on enough peanut sauce to cover all of it. Cover and place in fridge for 1 to 4 hours. (The more it sits, the more flavorful it gets)

Heat a small saucepan over medium heat. Pour in the marinated tofu and let sizzle, tossing every few minutes. Cook for about 10 minutes. You may need to add a bit more sauce according to your tastebuds.

Prepare a bed of the spinach and sliced cucumbers on plate and place the cooked tofu on top.

MAKES 1 SERVING

Per serving: 168 calories, 7 g protein, 16 g carbohydrates, 4 g total fat, 3 g dietary fiber, 280 mg sodium

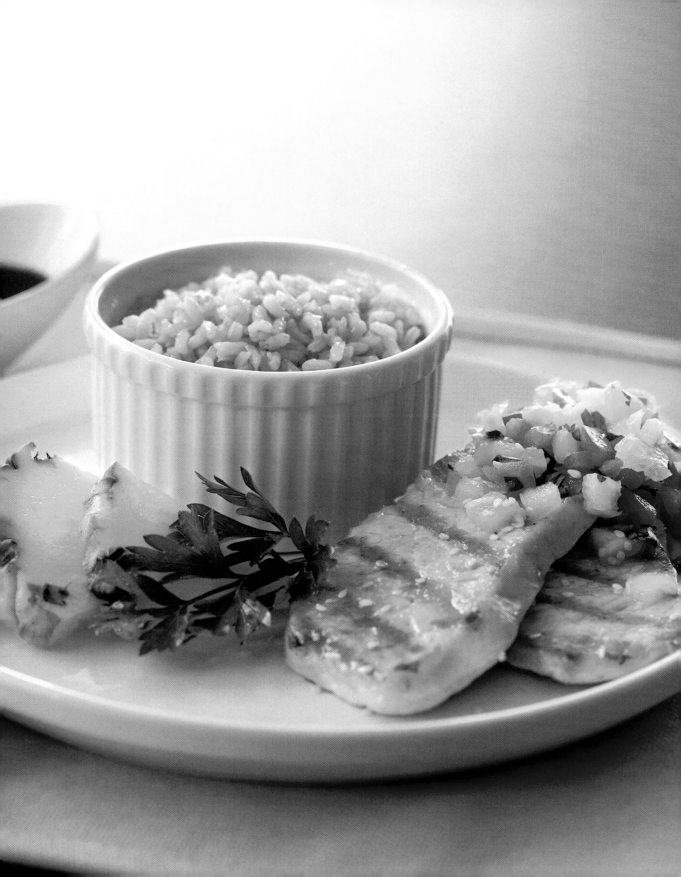

5-Minute Pork Chops

Okay, this looks like a "real" recipe that you might see on a cooking show but believe me, it's so easy, even I can do it! By the way, what's the very best ab exercise in the world? Walking away from the kitchen!

¼ cup + ⅛ cup natural honey

3 tablespoons soy sauce

4 cloves garlic, minced

4 pork loin chops, boneless, trimmed of excess fat, 4 ounces each

Uncle Ben's Ready Rice Whole Grain Brown

Mix the honey, soy sauce, and garlic in a bowl.

Toss the honey mix and pork into a resealable plastic storage bag and allow the meat to marinate several hours before the cooking time.

Throw all 4 chops on a George Foreman electric grill (no grease needed) or on any grill, tabletop or otherwise.

Cook 3 of the chops for 4 minutes. (We are undercooking these 3 just slightly so that when we warm them later in the week, they'll stay moist and not be overcooked!) Keep the fourth chop on the grill for a total of 5 minutes.

While you're cooking your pork chop, throw the pouch of rice in the microwave for 90 seconds.

Put ½ cup of the rice on your plate, toss a chop on top of it, cover and refrigerate the remaining chops and rice, and then get the heck out of the kitchen!

MAKES 4 SERVINGS

Per serving: 384 calories, 28 g protein, 47 g carbohydrates, 9 g total fat, 1 g dietary fiber, 56 mg sodium

Chocolate Shakeology Balls

OMG! I die! Seriously . . . I die! These are a mix between no-bake cookies and a frozen chocolate brownie. We keep dozens of these little balls of heaven in our freezer. They take a while to eat (when frozen) and they're filling. We fight over them, and all of our guests make a beeline for the freezer to see if we have any! Better than a protein bar, easier than a bag of processed junk, and healthier than most salads. Have these on hand at all times! *Warning:* Your family may need to have an intervention.

1 cup PB2 or Chocolate PB2 powdered peanut butter

½ cup natural peanut butter

1 cup quick oats

½ cup unsweetened applesauce

1 scoop Shakeology protein powder

Stevia, Truvía, or your choice of sweetener, to taste

In a large mixing bowl, throw in the peanut butters, oats, applesauce, protein powder, and sweetener. Mix together. The consistency will be pretty sticky and gooey.

Wet your hands in water, then roll the mixture into Ping-Pong-size balls.

Place on waxed paper or a plastic plate. Put in the freezer until firm, or enjoy right away if you can't resist!

MAKES 12

Per serving (2 cookies): 135 calories, 8 g protein, 13 g carbohydrates, 7 g total fat, 3 g dietary fiber, 13 mg sodium

Chalene's Guilt-Free Key Lime Protein Pie

It's yummy. Trust me.

1 cup Fage Total 0% Plain Greek Yogurt (or your favorite fat-free Greek-style yogurt)

Truvía or Stevia sweetener, to taste

1 pack True Lime or the juice of 1 fresh lime

Place the yogurt, sweetener, and lime juice in a bowl and mix! For an ice cream–like treat, set the bowl into the freezer for 25 minutes. Yummy!

MAKES 1 SERVING

Per serving: 131 calories, 20 g protein, 16 g carbohydrates, 0 g total fat, 0 g dietary fiber, 83 mg sodium

Chocolate Peanut Butter Nondairy Pudding

This is great as a late-night snack! I also freeze this in little cups—it kinda comes out like a poor man's frozen gelato.

- **½ cup unsweetened applesauce**
- **4 tablespoons Chocolate PB2 powdered peanut butter**
- **1 scoop Chocolate Shakeology protein powder (or your favorite protein powder)**
- **Truvía, Stevia, or your choice of sweetener, if needed**

Mix the applesauce, peanut butter, protein powder, and sweetener (if using) together in a bowl and *whoop whoop!!*

MAKES 1 SERVING

Per serving: 266 calories, 23 g protein, 44 g carbohydrates, 3 g total fat, 6 g dietary fiber, 142 mg sodium

Peanut Butter Chocolate Cheesecake

Chocolate and peanut butter lovers . . . get ready to fall over and faint when you eat this and then look at how good this is for you! This one recipe is worth the price of the whole book, if you ask me! (It's that good! It's that fast!)

- **1 cup Fage Total 0% Plain Greek Yogurt (or your favorite fat-free Greek-style yogurt)**
- **4 tablespoons Chocolate PB2 powdered peanut butter**
- **Truvía or Stevia sweetener, to taste**

Mix the yogurt, peanut butter, and sweetener all together and enjoy it!!

MAKES 1 SERVING

Per serving: 210 calories, 28 g protein (Whoa! That's better than most protein shakes!), 25 g carbohydrates, 2 g total fat, 2 g dietary fiber, 223 mg sodium

Pumpkin Pie Protein Pudding

Don't like yogurt? Feel free to make this with low-fat cottage cheese instead. The recipe makes one serving, but seriously, it's so low calorie, feel free to double it!

½ cup Fage Total 0% Plain Greek Yogurt (or your favorite fat-free Greek-style yogurt)

¼ cup canned organic pure pumpkin

Pinch of ground allspice

Dash of ground cinnamon

Pinch of Stevia or Truvía sweetener, to taste

Blend the yogurt, pumpkin, allspice, cinnamon, and sweetener in a bowl.

Grab your spoon and dig in. Divine.

MAKES 1 SERVING

Per serving: 81 calories, 11 g protein, 13 g carbohydrates, 0 g total fat, 3 g dietary fiber, 44 mg sodium

5-Minute Sweet Potato "Pie"

Sweet potatoes are what body builders and bikini models live on before a photo shoot! These spuds will make you lean but give you the much-needed energy and fiber you need! To cook a sweet potato in 5 minutes, use the individually wrapped ones in your produce isle. They say "microwaveable" on the plastic they're wrapped in. They turn out perfect and save tons of time!

1 small baked sweet potato

1 dash of ground nutmeg

1 teaspoon honey

Top the freshly warmed sweet potato with nutmeg and honey. Delish!

MAKES 1 SERVING

Per serving: 118 calories, 2 g protein, 28 g carbohydrates, 0 g total fat, 3 g dietary fiber, 10 mg sodium

ACKNOWLEDGMENTS

Brock and Cierra, you have inspired me to live my life according to my priorities. Nothing is more important than being with you. You have greatness within you and your unique gifts and belief in yourself will allow you to do great things and inspire others. You fill your father and me with love, pride, and purpose. Thank you for making me laugh and tipping me off on which hip-hop songs to download. Thanks for letting me be a mom who doesn't act her age and allowing me to interrogate your friends. Thank you for having an opinion but being thoughtful, self-motivated, and creative—so creative! Thank you for saying "I love you" to each other, even when you do it in your sarcastically silly voices. You can do anything!

To Bret, I love you. Together we have created two children beautiful inside and out. You have taught me resilience and what it means to grow stronger together. You still give me butterflies. Thanks for asking me to dance and convincing me to date a football player more than 20 years ago. I look forward to growing old and wrinkly with you as my partner in life and love.

I don't know what I would do without my sister Jenelle. You're the smartest, most dedicated, talented person I know who also finds me funny. We are so lucky to have what we share. To my younger brother, Bill, you are what every little girl needs in a father! (oh, and by the way, Jenelle and I decided when Mom and Dad get super old, they're moving in with you!) Thank you to my brother-in-law Rob for your unconditional support and for marrying an amazing woman like Dana! Dana, you are gold.

Monica Gray, you bless me with hilariousness everyday. No one makes me laugh or keeps me inspired like you do. I pray that everyone might find a friend like you. Mcayla Sarno, you are a quadruple threat. You're funny, a great dancer, a great singer, an awesome friend, and a doctor to boot.

I would never have acquired a taste for frog eating if it hadn't been for my mentor Brian Tracy. At every turn in my career for the past 16 years, I look to you for no-frills know-how. To Brendon Burchard who is more generous with knowledge than anyone I've ever met. You are what I call a passionate genius. My big brothers Carl Daikeler and Jon Congdon for believing in my dangerously unconventional approach to everything and for never giving up on me and giving me the opportunity to reach millions of people.

Shannon Welch, you helped me to create the book I was intended to write. You were encouraging and motivating and beyond patient when life unexpectedly threw a few curve balls. The team you assembled have talent beyond measure. Thank you to Chris Rhoads, Tiffany Bymaster, OC Films, Cassandra Delefortrie, Dan Mitchell, Sean Saint-Louis, Marie Crousillat, Nancy N. Bailey, Liz Krenos, Julia Van Tine, and Melissa Pearl for helping bring out the best in me.

The selfless heavy lifting awards go to Kevin Richards and Bret for doing all the technical, contractual, marketing, and planning that really makes this project a success. Kevin, thank you for your creativity, kind nature, and trusted friendship. To Denise Williams, thanks for your laugh, your expertise, and for always being my biggest cheerleader. Ben Gage, I'll never forget when you said, "I'll represent you until the moment you go Hollywood on me." You give Bret and me direction in more ways than you'll ever know. We are eternally grateful for your tell-it-like-it-is advice, keeping us grounded, and your belief in us. You are a trusted friend. Kristin, you are my life manager, my mind reader, my alarm clock, my crystal ball, my rock, and my friend. You inspire me away with your strength, resilience, and loyalty.

Lastly, I have to acknowledge all my Orange County students for pushing and supporting me along the journey. Your kick-butt attitudes and love means the world to me. You give me butterflies. To the millions of fans who have bought my workout DVDs (some of whom still haven't opened the package), I love ya and I'm here for you! You have greatness within you! Thank you for your trust and support. Now go create the life that you deserve!

ONLINE RESOURCES

Check it out. Here's a selection of Web sites I *love*. Visit these sites to learn more and to find some of the things, people, and places I recommend in *PUSH*!

Chalene Online

www.facebook.com/chalene
www.twitter.com/chalenejohnson
www.youtube.com/user/chalenejohnson
www.ustream.tv/chalenejohnson

People

BRIAN TRACY
www.briantracy.com

LORIE MARRERO, THE CLUTTER DIET
www.clutterdiet.com

ZIG ZIGLAR
www.ziglar.com

MONICA GRAY
www.partnerwithyourpartner.com

MICHAEL SENA
www.michaelsena.com

Support Groups

www.dailyburn.com
www.onlinefitnesslog.com
www.myyogaonline.com
www.beachbody.com
www.3fatchicks.com
www.30daypush.com

Mastermind Groups

www.lifehack.org

Fitness, Diet, Devices, Apps, and More!

BEACHBODY
www.beachbody.com

TEAM BEACHBODY
www.teambeachbody.com

LIVESTRONG
www.livestrong.com

CALORIE KING
www.calorieking.com

GET FIT BOOK
www.getfitbook.com

DISCOVERY HEALTH—BMR CALCULATOR
http://health.discovery.com

FIT WATCH—BMR CALCULAOR
www.fitwatch.com/qkcalc/bmr.html

SPARK PEOPLE
www.sparkpeople.com

FITBIT
www.fitbit.com

GOWEAR FIT
www.bodymedia.com

BODYBUGG
www.bodybugg.com.
http://bit.ly/CJBodybugg

BANDS/TUBING—SPRI DELUXE XERTUBE
www.spri.com

APPLE IPHONE , IPOD , ETC.
www.apple.com

AWESOME NOTES (PHONE APP)
http://bit.ly/CJAwesomeNote

GEORGE FOREMAN GRILL
www.georgeforemancooking.com

SMART SPIN STORAGE SYSTEM
www.amazon.com

EAT CLEANER FRUIT AND VEGETABLE SPRAY
www.eatcleaner.com

INDEX

Boldface page references indicate photographs. <u>Underscored</u> references indicate boxed text.